The Gout Diet & Cookbook

An Introduction to Low Purine Foods & Meals for People with Gout

Kenneth Martin

The Gout Diet & Cookbook

Copyright © 2017 by Kenneth Martin

ISBN: 978-1543247695

All rights reserved.

No part of this publication may be reproduced, distributed, or transmitted in any form or by any means, including photocopying, recording, or other electronic or mechanical methods, without the prior written permission of the publisher, except in the case of brief quotations embodied in critical reviews.

While the publisher and author have used their best efforts in preparing this book, they make no representations or warranties with respect to the accuracy or completeness of the content of this book. The material in this book is for informational purposes only. Since each individual situation is unique, you should use proper discretion, in consultation with a health-care practitioner, before undertaking the diet and strategies described in this book.

No warranty may be created or extended by the contributors/ authors, either implicitly or explicitly. The author and publisher expressly disclaim responsibility for any adverse effects that may result from the use or application of the information contained in this book.

Neither the publisher, nor contributors / authors shall be liable for any damages, including but not limited to special, incidental, consequential, or other damages.

The Gout Diet & Cookbook

Table of Contents

Introduction	iv
Chapter 1: What is Gout?	1
Chapter 2: Gout Diagnosis: The Importance of Getting It Right	4
Chapter 3: What is the Conventional Treatment of Gout?	7
Chapter 4: Lifestyle and Diet Changes	10
Chapter 5: Homeopathic / Home Remedies	14
Chapter 6: Breakfast	16
Chapter 7: Salads	26
Chapter 8: Soups & Appetizers	35
Chapter 10: Turkey	53
Chapter 11: Fish	61
Chapter 12: Meatless	69
Chapter 13: Desserts	77
Conclusion:	86

Introduction

Gout is horrible.

As a person who has Gout, I can safely say that it is no laughing matter. In fact, doctors say that next to childbirth and kidney stones, a gout attack is one of the most painful things a person can experience.

The "disease of kings" has now reached the masses. In the last half century alone, the condition has more than doubled. Along with obesity and hypertension, rates have steadily climbed. It now affects more than 8 million American adults and the numbers keep climbing. What is the culprit? Is it the fact that we are too sedentary and our food has become too processed?

In people who don't suffer from gout, eating purine rich foods such as red meat and shellfish can raise uric acid levels but their kidneys are efficient at eliminating it from the body in urine. However, people with gout actually have a defective mechanism for eliminating uric acid from the body – and this is thought to be a genetic predisposition.

Gout is a form of arthritis caused by high concentration of uric acid in the blood. This leads to the formation of tiny needle like crystals in the joints and kidneys (where they form kidney stones) and less commonly in other parts of the body including the spinal cord and the vocal chords. Gout is as painful as rheumatoid arthritis.

In any event, left untreated or uncontrolled, gout can form chalky lumps called tophi, which can severely damage joints, making walking and using the hands extremely painful. In extreme cases, joint replacements and even amputation is necessary.

Whether you need to take medicine for gout or not, you should ensure that you follow these simple rules of thumb to minimize gout:

- Limit alcoholic beverages and drinks sweetened with fruit sugar (fructose).
- Drink plenty of nonalcoholic beverages, especially water.
- Limit intake of foods high in purines, such as red meat, organ meats and seafood.
- Exercise regularly and lose weight. Keeping your body at a healthy weight reduces your risk of gout.

Having said that, this doesn't mean that your taste buds have to be affected. In the first part of this book we put into perspective just what gout is. In the latter part of the book we present a vast array of gout friendly food and meal options that covers everything from Breakfast to Dessert.

Eat up & enjoy.

Chapter 1: What is Gout?

Gout is a rheumatic condition that manifests itself through recurrent attacks of acute inflammatory arthritis—a red, tender, hot, swollen joint. Although gout can occur in any joint of your body and in multiple joints simultaneously, the joint at the base of the big toe, the metatarsal-phalangeal joint, is where it typically strikes.

Gout occurs when too much of a substance called uric acid builds up in the blood; this condition is also called hyperuricemia- elevated levels of uric acid in the blood. Uric acid can come from the breakdown of old cells and from certain foods and drinks. If too much uric acid is produced, or if it isn't properly excreted, it can form tiny crystals that are deposited in joints, tendons, and surrounding tissues. For this reason, gout is called a "crystal deposit disease." It may also present as tophi, kidney stones, or urate nephropathy – a kidney disease.

Essentially it is a breakdown of the metabolic process that controls the amount of uric acid in your blood. The stiffness and swelling are a result of excess uric acid forming crystals in your joints, and the pain associated with this disease is caused by your body's inflammatory response to the crystals.

What Are the Symptoms of Gout?

A gout attack, or "flare", usually strikes suddenly, and generally at night. Mysteriously, it often targets the large joint of your big toe. Your skin becomes red, inflamed, and overly sensitive. Even the light pressure of a bed sheet can become unbearable. A fever may also be present.

The pain associated with gout is often sudden and intense. Joints tend to swell, and can be warm to the touch. The skin around the joint may also take on a deep red or purple hue. People who have had gout for extended periods of time may develop nodules beneath the skin near joints; these are accumulations of uric acid crystals. Attacks can recur in the same joint over weeks, months or years, and repeated bouts of gout can damage the joint. Kidney damage can also occur.

With or without treatment, gout symptoms will usually go away within three to 10 days, and the next attack may not occur for months, or even years, if at all. Nonetheless, if more attacks occur, they tend to increase in frequency, become more severe, and last longer. Overtime, recurrent gout attacks can damage your joints and the surrounding areas.

This is why it's important to treat your gout as soon as possible, before it begins damaging your body permanently.

What Are the Causes of Gout?

Gout has a strong genetic component. The hallmark of gout is elevated blood levels of uric acid, a breakdown product of protein metabolism (a distinction should be made by a physician between true gout and pseudo gout, a similarly painful, arthritic condition that occurs when calcium pyrophosphate dehydrate crystals are deposited in a joint). Uric acid comes from the metabolism of purines, a subclass of proteins that are abundant in human tissues and such foods as organ meats, sardines, anchovies, mushrooms, asparagus and lentils.

Moreover, a number of drugs and supplements can increase uric acid levels in the blood and its tendency to form irritating crystals in joints. These include salicylates (the active component of aspirin), vitamin B3 (niacin), excess vitamin C and diuretics that may be prescribed for high blood pressure, edema or, cardiovascular disease. Others are Cyclosporine (used to prevent rejection of transplanted organs) and Levodopa for Parkinson's disease.

Excess alcohol consumption, being overweight, and exposure to lead in the environment also increase the risk of gout in genetically susceptible individuals. Other risk factors include dehydration and acid conditions of the blood that can result from serious infections, surgery or ketogenic weight loss diets (such as the Atkins diet). The genetic component should not be underestimated, however. It is possible to have high levels of uric acid and never develop gout.

Chapter 2: Gout Diagnosis: The Importance of Getting It Right

Many types of inflammatory arthritis, including gout, produce hot, stiff, inflamed, and painful joints. But just because someone has these symptoms doesn't necessarily mean that it's gout.

It is vital that a patient gets a proper diagnosis as Gout is a chronic disease and can lead to long-term damage.

Gout Diagnosis: Looking for Crystals

The first thing that doctors use to make an accurate diagnosis is a patient's history. Your age, sex, family history, weight, and diet are all risk factors for gout. Kidney and cardiovascular problems, as well as medications taken for these and other conditions, can also be associated with gout.

The true determinant, however, comes with a test to look for the hallmark sign of gout: uric acid crystals.

Visiting your doctor during an attack can ensure an accurate diagnosis. Drawing joint fluid during an acute attack so you can identify the uric acid crystals. The fluid is examined under a microscope with special filters so the crystals, if there are any, show up.

Bear in mind that even if crystals aren't seen in the fluid, gout can't be ruled out just yet. Further samples may be taken to see if there are crystals in the joints themselves, both those that are inflamed and others that don't appear affected. If tophi (harder, more permanent uric acid deposits) have developed, these can also be used to find uric acid, or urate crystals.

Taking fluid from swollen joints can rule out other problems, including inflammation due to infection and swelling caused by different types of crystals, such as those found in the very similar pseudo gout.

Gout Diagnosis: Looking for Hyperuricemia

Why can't a simple blood be used to diagnose gout? While most people will have elevated uric acid levels at some point during their disease, during a gout attack it's not unusual for those levels to be normal. Furthermore, levels of uric acid may also be checked in a urine sample.

However, you may not develop gout just because you have hyperuricemia. On the other hand, because people with chronic gout often have hyperuricemia when they don't have acute inflammation, blood tests may be used to monitor whether a medication is doing its job at bringing down uric acid levels.

Gout Diagnosis: Other Signs of Gout

Patients may have other physical signs of gout that last beyond the acute period. In addition to the tophi, which may develop underneath the skin — especially on the elbows and behind the ears, — uric acid may also cause kidney stones.

If tophi and perhaps kidney stones have developed, they indicate that gout has been present for a number of years, and the damage may be visible on an X-ray. The longer you go without treatment, the more likely you are to have permanent joint, and even kidney, damage. If you have hot, throbbing, almost unbearable pain in the big toe, contact your doctor. Even if the pain eases in a day or so, gout may be to blame.

In summary , the following tests to help diagnose gout may include:

- **Joint fluid test.** Your doctor may use a needle to draw fluid from your affected joint. When examined under the microscope, your joint fluid may reveal urate crystals.

- **Blood test.** Your doctor may recommend a blood test to measure the levels of uric acid and creatinine in your blood.

Remember, blood test results can be misleading, though. Some people have high uric acid levels, but never experience gout. And some people have signs and symptoms of gout, but don't have unusual levels of uric acid in their blood.

- **X-ray imaging.** Joint X-rays can be helpful to rule out other causes of joint inflammation.

- **Ultrasound.** Musculoskeletal ultrasound can detect urate crystals in a joint or in a tophus. This technique is more widely used in Europe than in the United States.

- **Dual energy CT scan.** This type of imaging can detect the presence of urate crystals in a joint, even when it is not acutely inflamed. This test is not used routinely in clinical practice due to the expense and is not widely available.

Chapter 3: What is the Conventional Treatment of Gout?

There is no known cure for gout, but it can be alleviated through a variety of conventional therapies and gout treatments. Physicians often prescribe non-steroidal anti-inflammatory drugs (NSAIDs) such as ibuprofen to keep inflammation and pain under control. Corticosteriods can have a similar affect; these are administered via pills or injections. There are also medicines that can lower levels of uric acid, the best known is probably allopurinol (Zyloprim). All of these measures should be used only as a last resort, as all carry the risk of significant side effects.

Medications to Treat Gout Attacks

Drugs used to treat acute attacks and prevent future attacks include:

- **Nonsteroidal anti-inflammatory drugs (NSAIDs).** NSAIDs include over-the-counter options such as ibuprofen (Advil, Motrin IB, others) and naproxen sodium (Aleve, others), as well as more-powerful prescription NSAIDs such as indomethacin (Indocin) or celecoxib (Celebrex).

Your doctor may prescribe a higher dose to stop an acute attack, followed by a lower daily dose to prevent future attacks.

NSAIDs carry risks of stomach pain, bleeding and ulcers.

- **Colchicine.** Your doctor may recommend colchicine (Colcrys, Mitigare), a type of pain reliever that effectively reduces gout pain. The drug's effectiveness is offset in most cases, however, by intolerable side effects, such as nausea, vomiting and diarrhea.

After an acute gout attack resolves, your doctor may prescribe a low daily dose of colchicine to prevent future attacks.

- **Corticosteroids.** Corticosteroid medications, such as the drug prednisone, may control gout inflammation and pain. Corticosteroids may be administered in pill form, or they can be injected into your joint.

Corticosteroids are generally reserved for people who can't take either NSAIDs or colchicine. Side effects of corticosteroids may include mood changes, increased blood sugar levels and elevated blood pressure.

Medications to Prevent Gout Complications

If you experience several gout attacks each year or if your gout attacks are less frequent but particularly painful, your doctor may recommend medication to reduce your risk of gout-related complications.

Options include:

- **Medications that block uric acid production.** Drugs called xanthine oxidase inhibitors, including allopurinol (Aloprim, Lopurin, Zyloprim) and febuxostat (Uloric), limit the amount of uric acid your body makes. This may lower your blood's uric acid level and reduce your risk of gout.

Side effects of allopurinol include a rash and low blood counts. Febuxostat side effects include rash, nausea and reduced liver function.

- **Medication that improves uric acid removal.** Probenecid (Probalan) improves your kidneys' ability to remove uric acid from your body. This may lower your uric acid levels and reduce your risk of gout, but the level of uric acid in your urine is increased. Side effects include a rash, stomach pain and kidney stones.

Chapter 4: Lifestyle and Diet Changes

Medications are the most proven, effective way to treat gout symptoms. However, making certain diet and lifestyle changes also may help, such as:

- Limiting alcoholic beverages and drinks sweetened with fruit sugar (fructose). Instead, drink plenty of nonalcoholic beverages, especially water.

- Limit intake of foods high in purines, such as red meat, organ meats and seafood.

- Exercising regularly and losing weight. Keeping your body at a healthy weight reduces your risk of gout.

High-Fructose Corn Syrup (HFCS)

Although gout is commonly blamed on eating too many high-purine foods, such as organ meats, anchovies, herring, asparagus and mushrooms, there is another clear culprit— high-fructose corn syrup.

Countless health problems have been linked to the consumption of high fructose corn syrup, not the least of which is gout. A recent study showed that consumption of sugar-sweetened soft drinks is strongly associated with an increased risk of developing gout.

The study, done by U.S. and Canadian researchers, indicated that men who drank two or more sugary soft drinks a day had an 85 percent higher risk of gout than those who drank less than one a month. In fact, the risk significantly increased among men who drank five to six servings of sugary soft drinks a week. Fruit juice and fructose-rich fruits, such as oranges and apples, also increased the risk

This makes sense on many levels, but first and foremost because fructose is known to inhibit the excretion of uric acid. Fructose also reduces the affinity of insulin for its receptor, which is the principle characteristic of type 2 diabetes. Furthermore, High Fructose Corn Syrup has been implicated in elevated blood cholesterol levels, and it has been found to inhibit the action of white blood cells in your immune system.

Many of the health conditions that HFCS causes, including high cholesterol and diabetes, also increase your risk of developing gout. Additionally, fructose converts more readily to fat than other sugars, making it a major risk factor for both diabetes and obesity -- another gout risk factor.

In a fructose metabolism study, it was noted that when two high-fructose breakfast drinks were consumed, the build-up of stored fat continued into the afternoon, during which time the quick conversion of fructose to fat remained active during digestion of the lunch meal. The study concluded that the higher the concentration of fructose in the diet, the higher the rate of fat conversion.

Frequently, fruit juices also have fructose added to them, and if you still believe that this is an acceptable form of sugar, think again. Fructose contains no beneficial enzymes, vitamins, minerals, or additional micronutrients. Instead, it actually leeches them from your body. Unbound fructose, found in large quantities in high fructose corn syrup, can also interfere with your heart's use of vital minerals such as magnesium, copper, and chromium.

Look At the Labels

You may think that avoiding fructose means just staying stay away from desserts and sweet drinks, but unfortunately there is more to it as fructose is hidden in many foods you would not even suspect. Names such as:: 'chicory,' 'inulin,' 'iso glucose,' 'glucose-fructose syrup,' 'dahlia syrup,' 'tapioca syrup,' 'glucose syrup,' 'corn syrup,' 'crystalline fructose,' and flat-out fraud 'fruit fructose,' or... 'agave'. Even processed meats and other foods you would never imagine contain high fructose corn syrup.

Limiting Alcohol is Crucial for Successful Gout Treatment

Gout is often seen in association with hypertension, excessive alcohol consumption, and coronary artery disease, so alcohol is a strong risk factor for this disease. In general, I believe alcohol should be reserved for people who have already achieved optimal wellness and therefore have their carbohydrates (sugars and grains) under control, and do not have disease conditions such as gout, diabetes, or other signs of ill health.

Although wine has been shown to have some health benefits, it may also increase your insulin levels, which is not only a risk factor for diabetes, but increased insulin levels have been linked with a shorter life span, in general. So it needs to be used cautiously, especially if you have gout. Most importantly for those suffering with gout, alcohol may raise the levels of uric acid in your blood, and therefore could even initiate a gout attack, so it's wise to limit the alcohol you drink, or eliminate it altogether.

Drink Water

Drink plenty of water to help flush the system. Dehydration is a major culprit of gout. To counter dehydration and minimize uric acid deposits in the joints drink 8, 8 oz glasses of water per day.

Exercise Can Dramatically Help

While exercise is not recommended while your joints are in pain or when it might cause further injury, once your gout is under control, exercise is needed as a necessary adjunct to a healthier lifestyle. Exercise will even help prevent further attacks by increasing circulation and normalizing your uric acids levels, which it does primarily by normalizing your insulin levels.

An exercise routine has other advantages as well. Studies have shown that it works as an effective antidepressant, strengthens your immune system so it can fight off diseases like cancer, and it can even improve insulin resistance and reverse pre-diabetic conditions.

Maintaining Ideal Body Weight is a Large Part of the Solution

It seems to me, one of the greatest risk factors for gout is obesity, or any excessive weight gain. Approximately half of all gout sufferers are overweight. Excess weight worsens gout because irritated nerve endings are further irritated by having to support and deal with extra weight. Furthermore, medical data shows a remarkably high prevalence of metabolic syndrome (heart disease and diabetes symptoms such as insulin resistance, abdominal obesity, hypertension, and high triglyceride levels) in gout sufferers.

Weight loss represents a safe method for reducing inflammatory states. Remember, gout is an inflammatory condition, and it is clear that losing weight, and keeping it off, will greatly improve your chances of avoiding further gout attacks.

Chapter 5: Homeopathic / Home Remedies

If gout treatments aren't working as well as you'd hoped, you may be interested in trying an alternative approach. Before trying such a treatment on your own, talk with your doctor — to weigh the benefits and risks and learn whether the treatment might interfere with your gout medication. Because there isn't a lot of research on alternative therapies for gout, in some cases the risks aren't known.

Certain foods have been studied for their potential to lower uric acid levels, including:

- **Coffee.** Studies have found an association between coffee drinking — both regular and decaffeinated coffee — and lower uric acid levels, though no study has demonstrated how or why coffee may have such an effect.

The available evidence isn't enough to encourage non coffee drinkers to start, but it may give researchers clues to new ways of treating gout in the future.

- **Vitamin C.** Supplements containing vitamin C may reduce the levels of uric acid in your blood. However, no studies have demonstrated that vitamin C affects the frequency or severity of gout attacks.

Talk to your doctor about what a reasonable dose of vitamin C may be. And don't forget that you can increase your vitamin C intake by eating more vegetables and fruits, especially oranges.

- **Cherries.** Cherries have been associated with lower levels of uric acid in studies, as well as a reduced number of gout attacks. Eating more cherries and drinking cherry extract may be a safe way to supplement your gout treatment, but discuss it with your doctor first.

- **Apple cider vinegar.** Helping to make the body more alkaline, apple cider vinegar has become a well-known proven solution for countless ailments, including gout. Try mixing 1-2 tablespoons of apple cider vinegar in 8 ounces of water. You can either drink it in one sitting or sip on it over time – try both methods and see which is more effective. This solution can reduce pain by 90% within a day or two.

- **Baking Soda.** Among other home remedies for gout is the use of baking soda. Mixing baking soda in water can effectively relieve pain almost instantly, though it may take 1-2 days. Mix 1/2 teaspoon baking soda in 8 oz. of water and drink it in one sitting. You may need to repeat this a few times a day, taking as much as 3 teaspoons total. Reduce the dose as the pain goes away. Note: The maximum recommended dose is 4 teaspoons throughout the day. Lastly, use caution if you suffer from hypertension, as baking soda may raise blood pressure when taken in larger amounts.
- **Bromelain/ Pineapples.** a compound that can be found in pineapples or in a supplement form. The enzymes within are frequently recommended for people with gout and have even been shown to have anti-cancer properties.

- **Beet juice.** Beet juice can help prevent acidosis and stimulates the liver to cleanse bile ducts.

- **Turmeric.** Turmeric has been gaining popularity in the last few years as a home remedy for gout. Use it to reduce inflammation and oxidative stress.

Chapter 6: Breakfast

Oatmeal Pancakes with Maple Fruit

Ingredients

- 3 medium bananas peeled and sliced
- ½ cup fresh blueberries
- ¼ maple syrup
- 2 teaspoons lemon juice
- ¼ teaspoon ground cinnamon
- 1 cup flour
- ½ cup quick cooking rolled oats
- ½ teaspoons baking powder
- ½ teaspoon baking soda
- 1/8 teaspoon salt
- 1 cup low-fat buttermilk or sour milk
- 1 egg, lightly beaten
- 1 tablespoon canola oil
- 1 tablespoon maple syrup
- 1 teaspoon vanilla

Directions

1. For the maple fruit, in a medium bowl stir together the bananas, blueberries, ¼ cup maple syrup, the lemon juice and cinnamon. Put aside.
2. In a large bowl, stir together flour, oats, baking powder, baking soda and salt. In a medium bowl, use a fork to combine buttermilk, egg, oil, the tablespoon of maple syrup and vanilla. Add the buttermilk mixture to the flour mixture. Stir until properly incorporated and moistened. Let stand for 10 minutes.
3. For each pancake, spoon 2 slightly rounded tablespoons of batter onto hot greased skillet or griddle. Spread to a 3 to 4 inch circle. Cook over medium heat for 1 to 2 minutes on

each side or until pancakes are golden brown. Turn over when edges are slightly dry and bottoms are browned. Serve warm topped with maple syrup.

Scrambled Eggs

Ingredients

- 8 eggs
- 1(5 ounce) can evaporated milk
- 2 tablespoons butter
- salt and pepper for taste

Directions

1. In a bowl, whisk the eggs and milk until combined.
2. In a skillet, heat butter until hot.
3. Add egg mixture; cook and stir over medium-low heat until eggs are completely set.
4. Season with salt and pepper.

Sunrise Fruit Salad

Ingredients

- ½ of an 8 ounce container of light cream cheese
- 6 ounce container of plain fat free Greek Yogurt
- 1 tablespoon honey
- 1 teaspoon finely shredded lemon peel
- 1 teaspoon finely shredded orange peel
- 1 medium orange, peeled and sectioned
- 3 medium kiwifruits, peeled and sliced
- 1 medium mango, seeded, peeled and cubed

- 1 cup of fresh blueberries

Directions

1. In a medium bowl, with an electric mixer set at medium beat the cream cheese until smooth. Beat in the the yogurt and honey until smooth. Then, stir in the orange and lemon peel.
2. Divide the mixture among 6 serving dishes. Top with fruit and serve immediately.

Corn Muffins

Ingredients

- Non-stick cooking spray
- 1 cup flour
- ¾ cup cornmeal
- ¼ cup sugar or substitute sweetener
- 2 ½ teaspoons baking powder
- ¾ teaspoon salt
- 2 beaten eggs
- 1 cup of fat-free milk
- ¼ cup of vegetable oil

Directions

1. Preheat the oven to 400 degrees. Coat twelve 2 ½ -inch muffin cups with cooking spray. In a medium bowl combine the flour, cornmeal, sugar, baking powder and salt. Set aside.
2. In a small bowl, combine eggs, milk and oil. Add this mixture to the flour mixture. Stir together until properly incorporated and moistened.
3. Spoon batter in to prepared muffin cups, filling each cup two-thirds full.
4. Bake about 15 minutes or until lightly browned. Serve warm.

Citrus Fruit Bowl

Ingredients

- 3 oranges peeled and slices crosswise
- 1 pink grapefruit peeled and sliced crosswise
- 2 tablespoons of honey
- 2 tablespoons crumbled fat-free feta cheese
- 1 tablespoon snipped fresh mint

Directions

1. Arrange the oranges and grapefruit slices in four shallow bowls. Drizzle with the honey; sprinkle with feta cheese and mint.
2. Serve chilled.

Eggs Benedict

Ingredients

- 4 slices Canadian bacon
- 1 teaspoon white vinegar
- 4 eggs
- 1 cup butter
- 3 egg yolks
- 1 tablespoon heavy cream
- 1 dash ground cayenne pepper
- ½ teaspoon salt
- 1 tablespoon lemon juice
- 4 whole wheat English muffins, split and toasted

Directions

1. In a skillet over medium-high heat, fry the Canadian bacon on each side until evenly browned.
2. Fill a large saucepan with about 3 inches water, and bring to a simmer. Pour in the vinegar. Carefully break the 4 eggs into the water, and cook 2 to 3 minutes, until whites are set but yolks are still soft. Remove eggs with a slotted spoon.

3. Meanwhile, melt the butter until bubbly in a small pan or in the microwave. Remove from heat before butter browns.
4. In a blender or large food processor, blend the egg yolks, heavy cream, cayenne pepper, and salt until smooth. Add half of the hot butter in a thin steady stream, slow enough so that it blends in at least as fast as you are pouring it in. Blend in the lemon juice using the same method, then the remaining butter.
5. Place open English muffins onto serving plates. Top with 1 slice Canadian bacon and 1 poached egg. Drizzle with the cream sauce, and serve at once.

Cherry Pecan Muffins

Ingredients

- 2 cups all-purpose flour
- ½ teaspoon salt
- 1 teaspoons baking powder
- ½ teaspoon baking soda
- ¼ teaspoon nutmeg
- 2 large eggs
- 1/3 cup vegetable oil
- ¼ cup milk
- ½ teaspoon almond extract
- 1/3 brown sugar
- 1 cup sour cream
- 1 10 ounce jar of maraschino cherries, drained and chopped
- 2/3 cup pecans, chopped

For the topping:

- ¼ cup all-purpose flour
- ¼ cup brown sugar
- ½ teaspoon of cinnamon
- 2 tablespoons butter

Directions

1. Preheat the oven to 425 degrees. In a medium bowl, mix the flour, salt, baking powder, baking soda, and nutmeg. In another bowl, whisk two large eggs. Add the oil, milk, extract, brown sugar, and sour cream. Blend well. Stir in the cherries and nuts. With a spatula, mix the dry ingredients into the liquid mixture. Stir until just combined.
2. Spoon the batter into 10 to 12 well-greased muffin tins. Ten muffins will give you large, nicely-domed muffins. Fill any unused muffins cups half full of water. 4. In a small bowl, mix the flour, brown sugar, and cinnamon. Cut the butter in with a pastry knife until you have a coarse mixture. Spoon the topping onto the muffins before baking.
3. Bake for eight minutes at 425 degrees. Reduce the temperature to 350 degrees and continue baking for another 6 to 10 minutes or until they test done with a toothpick. Let the muffins sit in the tins for a few and then place on wire racks to cool.

Baked Apple Oatmeal

Ingredients

- 2 2/3 cups old-fashioned oats
- ½ cup raisins
- 4 cups milk
- 1/3 cup packed brown sugar
- 2 tablespoons butter or margarine, melted
- 1 teaspoon ground cinnamon
- ¼ teaspoon salt
- 2 medium apples, chopped (2 cups)
-

Directions

1. 1 Heat oven to 350°F. In 2-quart casserole, mix oats, raisins, 4 cups milk, the brown sugar, butter, cinnamon, salt and apples.
2. 2 Bake uncovered 40 to 45 minutes or until most liquid is absorbed. Top with walnuts. Serve with additional milk.

Zucchini & Eggs

Ingredients

- 4 eggs, lightly beaten
- 2 tablespoons grated Parmesan cheese
- 2 tablespoons olive oil
- 1 zucchini, sliced 1/8- to ¼-inch thick
- garlic powder or salt
- ground black pepper to taste

Directions

1. Stir the eggs and Parmesan cheese together in a bowl; set aside.
2. Heat the olive oil in a large skillet over medium-high heat; cook the zucchini in the hot oil until softened and lightly browned, about 7 minutes. Season the zucchini with garlic powder, salt, and pepper. Reduce heat to medium; pour the egg mixture into the skillet. Cook, stirring gently, for about 3 minutes.
3. Remove the skillet from the heat and cover. Keep covered off the heat until the eggs set, about 2 minutes more and serve.

Pumpkin Pancakes

Ingredients

- 1 ¼ cups all-purpose flour
- 2 tablespoons sugar
- 2 teaspoons baking powder
- ½ teaspoon cinnamon
- ½ teaspoon ginger
- ½ teaspoon nutmeg
- ½ teaspoon salt
- 1 pinch clove
- 1 cup 1% low-fat milk
- 6 tablespoons canned pumpkin puree
- 2 tablespoons melted butter
- 1 egg

Directions

1. Whisk flour, sugar, baking powder, spices and salt in a bowl.
2. In a separate bowl whisk together milk, pumpkin, melted butter, and egg.
3. Fold mixture into dry ingredients.
4. Spray or grease a skillet and heat over medium heat: pour in 1/4 cup batter for each pancake.
5. Cook pancakes about 3 minutes per side. Serve with butter and syrup. Makes about six 6-inch pancakes.

Cornflakes with Berries

Ingredients

1. 2 cups cornflakes
2. 1 cup 1% low-fat milk
3. 1 cup berries, fresh or frozen, thawed

Directions

1. Place cornflakes in a small bowl.
2. Top with milk and berries and serve.

Berry Breakfast Quinoa

Ingredients:

- ¼ cup milk
- 2 containers (6 oz each) 99% Fat Free French vanilla, strawberry or peach yogurt
- 4 teaspoons chia seed
- 1 cup cooled cooked quinoa (1/4 cup uncooked)
- 2 cups fresh fruit (mixed berries or chopped peaches)
- ¼ cup coarsely chopped toasted almonds or pecans
- 1/8 teaspoon ground cinnamon

Directions:

1. In medium bowl, stir together milk, yogurt and chia seed until blended. Evenly divide mixture among 4 glasses. Spoon 1/4 cup cooled cooked quinoa on top of yogurt layer on each.
2. Top each with a layer of fruit and almonds. Sprinkle with cinnamon. Let stand 5 minutes, or cover and refrigerate overnight.

Banana-Blueberry Smoothie

Ingredients:

- 1 cup milk
- 1 cup Cheerios cereal

- 1 ripe banana, cut into chunks
- 1 cup fresh blueberries
- 1 cup ice
- Garnishes, If Desired
- Banana slices
- Additional cereal

Directions:

1. In blender, place Smoothie ingredients. Cover; blend on high speed about 30 seconds or until smooth.
2. Pour into 2 glasses. Garnish as desired. Serve immediately.

Cherry Strawberry Smoothie

Ingredients:

- 2 containers (5.3 oz each) honey Greek yogurt
- 1 ½ cups frozen organic cherries
- ½ cup frozen organic strawberries
- 1 cup milk

Directions:

1. In blender, place all ingredients. Cover and blend on high speed about 1 minute or until smooth.
2. Pour into 3 glasses. Serve immediately.

Chapter 7: Salads

Zesty Garden Salad

Ingredients

- 1 teaspoon Dijon mustard
- 1 sprig fresh dill, chopped (optional)
- 1 tablespoon chopped green onion
- 2 tablespoons shredded Cheddar cheese
- ½ cup sweet corn kernels
- ½ cup sugar snap peas
- 1/3 cup frozen shelled edamame (optional)
- 2 cups iceberg lettuce
- 1 pinch salt and pepper

Directions

1. Stir the Dijon mustard, dill, green onion, Cheddar cheese, corn, peas, and edamame in a bowl until evenly combined.
2. Stir in the iceberg lettuce, season to taste with salt and pepper, and toss to mix.

Greek Salad

Ingredients

- 1 head romaine lettuce- rinsed, dried and chopped
- 1 red onion, thinly sliced
- 1 (6 ounce) can pitted black olives
- 1 green bell pepper, chopped
- 1 red bell pepper, chopped
- 2 large tomatoes, chopped

- 1 cucumber, sliced
- 1 cup crumbled feta cheese
- 6 tablespoons olive oil
- 1 teaspoon dried oregano
- 1 lemon, juiced
- ground black pepper

Directions

1. In a large salad bowl, combine the Romaine, onion, olives, bell peppers, tomatoes, cucumber and cheese.
2. Whisk together the olive oil, oregano, lemon juice and black pepper.
3. Pour dressing over salad, toss and serve.

Cherry Tomato Corn Salad

Ingredients

- 1/4 cup minced fresh basil
- 3 tablespoons olive oil
- 2 teaspoons lime juice
- 1 teaspoon sugar
- 1/2 teaspoon salt
- 1/4 teaspoon pepper
- 2 cups frozen corn, thawed
- 2 cups cherry tomatoes, halved
- 1 cup chopped seeded peeled cucumber

Directions

1. In a jar with a tight-fitting lid, combine the basil, oil, lime juice, sugar, salt and pepper; shake well.
2. In a large bowl, combine the corn, tomatoes and cucumber.

3. Drizzle with dressing and toss to coat. Refrigerate until serving.

Summer Watermelon Salad

Ingredients

- ¼ cup balsamic vinegar
- 1 tablespoon Dijon mustard
- 1 tablespoon chopped garlic
- ½ teaspoon salt
- ½ teaspoon freshly ground black pepper
- ¾ cup olive oil
- 3 cups 2-inch cubes watermelon
- 1 cup crumbled feta cheese
- ½ red onion, sliced very thin
- coarsely ground black pepper for taste

Directions

1. Mix the vinegar and Dijon mustard in a bowl. Stir the garlic, salt, and pepper into the mixture. Slowly stream the olive oil into the dressing while whisking vigorously. Place the dressing in the refrigerator until ready to use.
2. Combine the watermelon, feta cheese, and red onion in a large bowl; toss lightly to mix. Season with the coarsely ground black pepper.
3. Pour about half the dressing over the salad; gently toss to coat. Refrigerate the salad at least 30 minutes. Drizzle the remaining dressing over the salad just before serving.

Asian Tofu Salad

Ingredients

- ¼ cup reduced sodium soy sauce
- ¼ cup of sweet chili sauce
- 1 tablespoon creamy peanut butter
- 1 clove garlic, minced
- 1 teaspoon grated fresh ginger
- 1 16 to 18 ounce package firm water packed tofu
- 1 teaspoon toasted sesame oil
- 4 cups shredded romaine lettuce
- 1 ½ cups chopped, peeled jicama
- 1 medium red sweet pepper, seeded and thinly sliced
- 1 cup coarsely shredded carrots
- 2 tablespoons unsalted dry-roasted peanuts
- 2 tablespoons snipped fresh cilantro

Directions

1. In a small bowl, whisk together soy sauce, chili sauce, peanut butter, garlic and ginger. Pat tofu dry with paper towels. Cut tofu crosswise into 12 slices. Place tofu in a 2-quart rectangular baking dish. Drizzle with 3 tablespoons of the soy sauce mixture, turning to coat the tofu. Let marinate at room temperature for 30 minutes, turning tofu occasionally. Set aside the remaining soy sauce mixture for dressing.
2. In a very large non-stick skillet heat sesame oil over medium-high heat. Remove tofu from the marinade. Add remaining marinade to skillet. Add the tofu slices. Cook for 5 – 6 minutes or until lightly browned, turning once halfway through cooking.
3. In a large bowl, combine lettuce, jicama, sweet pepper, and carrots. Divide among six serving plates. Top with tofu,

peanuts and cilantro. Serve with the reserved dressing mixture.

Apple-Tomato Salad

Ingredients

- 2 cups green leaf lettuce, torn into bite size pieces
- 2 cups arugula
- 1 cup cherry tomatoes, halved
- 1 medium Fuji apple or Granny Smith apple, halved and thinly sliced
- ¼ of a medium red onion, thinly sliced
- 2 tablespoons crumbled blue cheese
- 4 teaspoons chopped pecans,
- 2 tablespoons of cider vinegar
- 4 teaspoons of olive oil
- 1 tablespoon honey
- 1/8 teaspoon salt
- 1/8 teaspoon black pepper

Directions

1. Arrange leaf lettuce, arugula, tomatoes, apple and red onion on four salad plates. Sprinkle with blue cheese and pecans.
2. For the dressing, in a screw top jar combine vinegar, olive oil, honey, salt and pepper. Cover and shake well. Drizzle dressing over salads.

Orange & Duck Confit Salad

Ingredients

- 1 tablespoon sherry vinegar
- 4 blood oranges, divided (3 sectioned, about 1 cup; 1 juiced, about 1/4 cup)

- 1 teaspoon Dijon mustard
- 1 tablespoon olive oil
- ¼ teaspoon salt
- ¼ teaspoon pepper
- 1 small duck confit leg (5-6 ounces), shredded, skin, fat, and bones discarded (about 3/4 cup)
- 6 cups mixed winter salad greens (such as romaine, escarole, and spinach)
- ¼ cup skinned chopped hazelnuts, toasted

Directions

1. In a small bowl, combine vinegar, orange juice, mustard, and oil, whisking well. Whisk in salt and pepper.
2. In a large bowl, combine shredded duck, salad greens, hazelnuts, and orange sections. Drizzle with vinaigrette; serve.

Jicama Radish Slaw

Ingredients

- ¼ cup snipped cilantro
- 2 tablespoons rice vinegar
- 2 tablespoons toasted sesame oil
- ¼ teaspoon salt
- ¼ crushed red pepper
- ½ of a medium jicama, peeled and cut into thin match-stick size pieces (about three cups)
- ¾ cup radishes, trimmed and thinly sliced
- ½ cup julienne or packaged coarsely shredded fresh carrot
- 2 green onions, cut into 2 inch pieces and thinly sliced lengthwise
- Lime wedges (optional)

Directions

1. In a large bowl, whisk together cilantro, vinegar, oil, salt and crushed red pepper. Add jicama, radishes, carrot and green onions. Toss to coat.
2. Serve immediately. If desired, garnish with the lime wedges.

Grandma's Potato Salad

Ingredients

- 2 potatoes
- 1 sweet potato
- 4 eggs
- 2 stalks celery, chopped
- ½ onion, chopped
- ¾ cup mayonnaise
- 1 tablespoon prepared mustard
- 1 teaspoon salt
- 1 ½ teaspoons ground black pepper

Directions

1. Bring a large pot of salted water to a boil. Add potatoes and cook until tender but still firm, about 30 minutes. Drain, cool, peel and chop.
2. Place eggs in a saucepan and cover with cold water. Bring water to a boil. Cover, remove from heat, and let eggs stand in hot water for 10 to 12 minutes. Remove from hot water; cool, peel and chop.
3. Combine the potatoes, eggs, celery and onion. Whisk together the mayonnaise, mustard, salt and pepper. Add to potato mixture, toss well to coat. Refrigerate and serve chilled.

Winter Fruit Waldorf Salad

Ingredients:

- 2 medium unpeeled red apples, diced
- 2 medium unpeeled pears, diced
- ½ cup thinly sliced celery
- ½ cup golden raisins
- ½ cup chopped dates
- ¼ cup gluten-free mayonnaise or salad dressing
- ¼ cup 99% Fat Free orange crème yogurt (from 6-oz container)
- 2 tablespoons frozen orange juice concentrate
- 8 cups shredded lettuce
- Walnut halves, if desired

Directions:

1. In large bowl, mix apples, pears, celery, raisins and dates.
2. In small bowl, mix mayonnaise, yogurt and juice concentrate until well blended. Add to fruit; toss to coat. (Salad can be refrigerated up to 1 hour.) Serve on lettuce. Garnish with walnut halves.

Quinoa and Vegetable Salad

Ingredients:

- 1 cup uncooked quinoa
- 2 tablespoons fresh lemon juice
- 2 tablespoons olive oil
- 2 tablespoons chopped fresh basil
- 1 can (15 oz) gluten-free garbanzo beans, drained, rinsed

- 1 can (15.25 oz) gluten-free whole kernel sweet corn, drained
- 1 can (14.5 oz) gluten-free diced tomatoes, drained
- 1 cup chopped red bell pepper
- 1/3 cup quartered pitted olives
- ½ cup crumbled gluten-free feta cheese

Directions:

1. Rinse quinoa under cold water 1 minute; drain. Cook quinoa as directed on package; drain. Cool completely, about 30 minutes.
2. Meanwhile, in small nonmetal bowl, place lemon juice, oil and basil; mix well. Set aside for dressing.
3. In large bowl, gently toss cooked quinoa, beans, corn, tomatoes, bell pepper and olives. Pour dressing over quinoa mixture; toss gently to coat. Serve immediately or refrigerate 1 to 2 hours before serving.

Chapter 8: Soups & Appetizers

Caprese Appetizer

Ingredients

- 20 grape tomatoes
- 10 ounces mozzarella cheese, cubed
- 2 tablespoons extra virgin olive oil
- 2 tablespoons fresh basil leaves, chopped
- 1 pinch salt
- 1 pinch ground black pepper
- 20 toothpicks

Directions

1. Toss tomatoes, mozzarella cheese, olive oil, basil, salt, and pepper together in a bowl until well coated.
2. Skewer one tomato and one piece of mozzarella cheese on each toothpick.

Home-Style Potato Soup

Ingredients

- 3 medium potatoes (about 1 pound)
- 1 ¾ cups chicken broth (from 32-ounce carton)
- 2 medium green onions with tops
- 1 ½ cups milk
- ¼ teaspoon salt
- 1/8 teaspoon pepper
- 1/8 teaspoon dried thyme leaves

Directions

1. Peel the potatoes, and cut into large pieces.
2. Heat the chicken broth and potatoes to boiling in the saucepan over high heat, stirring occasionally with a fork to make sure potatoes do not stick to the saucepan. Once mixture is boiling, reduce heat just enough so mixture bubbles gently. Cover and cook about 15 minutes or until potatoes are tender when pierced with a fork.
3. While the potatoes are cooking, peel and thinly slice the green onions. If you have extra onions, wrap them airtight and store in the refrigerator up to 5 days.
4. When the potatoes are done, remove the saucepan from the heat, but do not drain. Break the potatoes into smaller pieces with the potato masher or large fork. The mixture should still be lumpy.
5. Stir the milk, salt, pepper, thyme and onions into the potato mixture. Heat over medium heat, stirring occasionally, until hot and steaming, but do not let the soup boil.

Gazpacho

Ingredients

- 1 hothouse cucumber. halved and seeded, but not peeled
- 2 red bell peppers, cored and seeded
- 4 plum tomatoes
- 1 red onion
- 2 garlic cloves, minced
- 3 cups tomato juice
- ¼ cup white wine vinegar
- ¼ cup olive oil
- ½ tablespoon salt

- 1 teaspoon freshly ground black pepper

Directions

1. Roughly chop the cucumbers, bell peppers, tomatoes, and red onions into 1-inch cubes.
2. Put each vegetable separately into a food processor fitted with a steel blade and pulse until it is coarsely chopped.
3. Once each vegetable is processed, combine them in a large bowl and add the garlic, tomato juice, vinegar, olive oil, salt, and pepper. Mix well and chill before serving.

Mint Ginger Sweet Potato Soup

Ingredients

- 1 tablespoon olive oil
- 2 medium-large sweet potatoes peeled, chopped, and pureed
- 1 clove garlic
- 1 teaspoon ginger
- 1/3 teaspoon turmeric
- 4 diced mint leaves
- 2 cups vegetable broth

Directions

1. Pour olive oil into food processor.
2. Add the washed, peeled and pieces of sweet potato into the food processor with the oil.
3. Add garlic clove to the food processor.
4. Add the ginger turmeric.
5. Wash, dry, and chop mint leaves.
6. Puree.
7. Pour into medium sized pot or Dutch oven.

8. Add broth.
9. Let sit over medium heat for 25-30 minutes.

Vegetables & Hummus

Ingredients

- ¾ cup mixed vegetables, such as baby carrots, cherry tomatoes and red bell pepper slices
- 1 (15.5 ounce) can garbanzo beans (chickpeas), drained 1/3 cup pitted Spanish Manzanilla olives
- 1 teaspoon minced garlic
- 3 tablespoons olive oil
- 2 tablespoons lemon juice
- 1 ½ teaspoons chopped fresh basil
- 1 teaspoon cilantro leaves
- salt and pepper

Directions

1. Wash vegetables and a slice them into bitable sizes.
2. Place garbanzo beans, olives, and garlic into the bowl of a blender or food processor. Pour in olive oil and lemon juice; season with basil, cilantro, salt, and pepper.
3. Cover and puree until smooth.
4. Arrange vegetables on a platter.
5. Dip into hummus and eat.

Carrot Soup

Ingredients

- 2 bags (1 lb each) ready-to-eat baby-cut carrots

- 2 large onions, chopped (about 2 cups)
- 5 ¼ cups chicken broth (from two 32-oz cartons)
- ½ teaspoon salt
- ½ cup whipping cream
- ½ cup orange juice
- 3 tablespoons packed brown sugar
- 2 tablespoons grated gingerroot
- ¼ teaspoon white pepper
- Fresh orange slices, quartered, if desired
- Fresh Italian parsley, if desired

Directions

1. Spray 4- to 5-quart slow cooker with cooking spray. In cooker, mix carrots, onions, broth and salt.
2. Cover; cook on Low heat setting 8 to 10 hours.
3. Pour 4 cups of the soup mixture to blender; add half each of the whipping cream, orange juice, brown sugar, gingerroot and pepper. Cover and blend until smooth; return to cooker. Blend remaining soup mixture with remaining half of ingredients; return to cooker.
4. Increase heat setting to High. Cover; cook 15 to 20 minutes longer or until hot. Garnish individual servings with an orange quarter and parsley.

<u>Deviled Eggs</u>

Ingredients

- 12 eggs 1 jalapeno pepper, minced
- 1 habanero peppers, seeded and minced
- ¼ cup mayonnaise
- 1 teaspoon yellow mustard
- 1/8 teaspoon paprika

Directions

1. Place the eggs into a saucepan in a single layer, and fill with water to cover the eggs by at least 1 inch. Bring the water to a boil over high heat. Cover, and remove from the heat; let the eggs stand in the hot water for 15 minutes. Pour out the hot water, then cool the eggs under cold running water in the sink. Peel.
2. Cut the cooled eggs in half lengthwise. Remove the yolks, and place them into a mixing bowl along with the jalapeno, habanero, mayonnaise, and mustard; mash together until smooth. Transfer the yolk mixture to a pastry bag, and decoratively squeeze into the white halves. Sprinkle with paprika to garnish.

Kale & Tofu

Ingredients

- 3 oz. fresh kale leaves
- 3 oz. firm tofu cubes
- Olive oil for drizzling
- No-salt seasoning

Directions

1. Prepare baking tray and preheat oven to 400.
2. Layout individual kale leaves, drop one tofu cube in the center. Fold leaf ends over tofu cube and flip.
3. Drizzle with olive oil and seasoning Bake 18-22 minutes.

Roasted Garlic & Cauliflower Soup

Ingredients

- 1 large head cauliflower (about 2 ½ lb.)
- 4 ½ teaspoons olive oil
- 1 ½ teaspoons kosher salt
- 3 garlic cloves, divided & unpeeled
- 3 cups chicken broth
- 1 cup 2% reduced-fat milk
- ½ cup grated Parmesan cheese
- Freshly ground black pepper
- Garnishes: olive oil, pomegranate seeds, fresh thyme leaves

Directions

1. Preheat oven to 425 °. Cut cauliflower into 2-inch florets; toss with olive oil and 1/ 2 tsp. salt. Arrange florets in a single layer on a jelly-roll pan. Wrap garlic cloves in aluminum foil, and place on jelly-roll pan with cauliflower.
2. Bake at 425 ° for 30 to 40 minutes or until cauliflower is golden brown, tossing cauliflower every 15 minutes.
3. Transfer cauliflower to a large Dutch oven. Unwrap garlic, and cool 5 minutes. Peel garlic, and add to cauliflower. Add stock, and bring to a simmer over medium heat; simmer, stirring occasionally, 5 minutes. Let mixture cool 10 minutes.
4. Process cauliflower mixture, in batches, in a blender until smooth, stopping to scrape down sides as needed.
5. Return cauliflower mixture to Dutch oven; stir in milk, cheese, and remaining 1 tsp. salt. Cook over low heat, stirring occasionally, 2 to 3 minutes or until thoroughly heated. Add pepper for taste.

Spinach and Potato Soup

Ingredients

- 2 cloves garlic, minced

- ½ cup chopped onion
- ½ teaspoon salt
- ¼ teaspoon black pepper
- 2 teaspoons olive oil
- 4 cups unsalted chicken stock
- 3 cups coarsely chopped yellow potatoes
- 5 ounces packaged fresh baby spinach (about 6 cups)
- 2 teaspoons snipped fresh rosemary or ½ teaspoon dried rosemary, crushed
- 2 6 ounce containers plain reduced-fat Greek Yogurt
- ½ cup chopped reduced-sodium ham (2 ½ ounces)
- ¼ chopped toasted almonds

Directions

1. In a large saucepan cook onion, garlic, salt and pepper in a hot oil over medium heat for 3 to 4 minutes or until onion is tender. Add 3 cups of chicken stock and potatoes. Bring to boiling; reduce heat. Cover and simmer for 15 to 20 minutes or until potatoes are tender.
2. Meanwhile, in a food processor/ blender combine half of the spinach and rosemary and ½ cup of the remaining stock. Cover and process or blend until smooth. Add blended spinach mixture to saucepan. Repeat with remaining spinach, rosemary and ½ cup stock; add to saucepan. Stir in ham and heat through making sure not to boil. To serve, ladle soup into bowls and top with almonds.

Egg Drop Soup

Ingredients

- Nonstick cooking spray
- 1 egg roll wrapper, cut in thin 1 to 1 ½ inch long strips
- 6 cups low sodium chicken broth

- 4 teaspoons reduced sodium soy sauce
- 1 clove garlic, minced
- ¼ teaspoon ground white pepper
- ½ cup frozen baby sweet peas
- 8 teaspoons cornstarch
- 4 eggs
- 2 green onions, bias sliced

Directions

1. Preheat oven to 375F. Lightly coat baking sheet with cooking spray. Place egg roll wrapper strips on prepared baking sheet. Lightly coat strips with cooking spray. Bake 6 to 7 minutes or until lightly browned and crisp, stirring once after 3 minutes; set aside.
2. In a large saucepan combine 5 cups of the broth, the soy sauce, garlic and pepper. Bring to boiling.
3. Add the peas to the boiling broth, then return to boiling
4. Stir cornstarch into remaining 1 cup of broth; stir into soup. Reduce heat. Cook and stir until slightly thickened and bubbly; cook and stir for two minutes more. Remove from heat. Place eggs in a liquid measuring cup; use a fork to beat eggs. While gently stirring the broth, pour eggs in a thin stream into soup. The eggs will form fine shreds.
5. To serve. Ladle the soup into bowls. Garnish individual servings with green onions. Serve with the crisp egg roll wrapper strips.

Veggie French Bread Pizza

Ingredients

- 1 loaf French bread
- 1 cup pizza sauce
- 1 to 2 cups shredded mozzarella cheese
- 1 4 ounce can sliced mushrooms, drained

- 1 16 ounce can artichoke hearts, drained
- ½ large green pepper, sliced
- ½ large red or yellow pepper, sliced
- ½ cup chopped red onion
- 1 2 ounce can sliced black olives, drained
- black pepper to taste

Directions

1. Pre-heat oven to 350 F Slice Loaf in half, length-wise, and spread each half with equal amounts of ingredients. Sprinkle lightly with black pepper.
2. Bake for 7 to 10 minutes, or until cheese melts.
3. To serve, slice each half into fourths.

Chapter 9: Chicken

Spice Rubbed Roast Chicken

Ingredients

- 2 tablespoons snipped fresh cilantro
- 2 teaspoons finely shredded orange peel
- ½ teaspoon salt
- ½ teaspoon ground coriander
- ½ teaspoon ground ginger
- ¼ teaspoon black pepper
- ¼ teaspoon ground allspice
- ¼ teaspoon crushed red pepper
- 1 3 ½ to 4 pound whole roasting chicken

Directions

1. Preheat oven to 375 degrees. In a small bowl, combine the 2 tablespoons cilantro, the orange peel, salt, coriander, ginger, black pepper, allspice and crushed red pepper. Rinse chicken

body cavity; remove any excess fat from cavity. Dry the chicken with paper towels.
2. Using your fingers, loosen the chicken skin from breast meat and drumsticks. Spoon cilantro mixture under the skin, rubbing it evenly over the breast and drumstick meat. Skewer neck skin of chicken to back; tie legs to tail. Twist wing tips under back. Place chicken, breast side up, on a rack in a shallow roasting pan. Insert an ovenproof meat thermometer into the center of an inside thigh muscle, making sure the tip does not touch bone.
3. Roast, uncovered for 1 ½ hours or until drumsticks move easily in their sockets and chicken is no longer pink. Cover and let stand for 15 minutes before serving. Remove skin and discard as you carve chicken.

Oven-Fried Parmesan Chicken

Ingredients

- 2 eggs beaten
- ¼ cup fat-free milk
- ¾ cup grated Parmesan cheese
- ¾ fine dry bread crumbs
- 2 teaspoons dried and crushed oregano
- 1 teaspoon paprika
- ¼ teaspoon black pepper
- 12 meaty chicken pieces (drumsticks, thighs, breast halves skinned) about 5 ½ total
- ¼ cup melted butter
- Lemon wedges (optional)

Directions

1. Preheat oven to 375 degrees. Grease two large shallow baking pans; set aside. In a bowl combine egg and milk. In a

shallow dish, combine Parmesan, bread crumbs, oregano, paprika and pepper.
2. Dip chicken pieces into egg mixture. Arrange chicken pieces in prepared baking pans, making sure pieces do not touch. Drizzle chicken with the melted butter.
3. Bake, uncover, for 45- 55 minutes until chicken is tender and no longer pink. Do not turn the chicken pieces during baking. You may sprinkle with fresh Oregano. Serve with lemon wedges.

Chicken Ragout

Ingredients

- 8 chicken thighs 3 ½ pounds total, skinned
- 2 14.5 ounce cans no salt added diced tomatoes, drained
- 3 cups 1 inch carrot slice or baby carrots
- 1 large onion cut into wedges (1 cup)
- 1/3 cup reduced sodium chicken broth
- 2 tablespoons white wine vinegar
- 1 teaspoon dried rosemary, crushed
- 1 teaspoon dried thyme, crushed
- ¼ teaspoon black pepper
- 8 ounces fresh button mushrooms, sliced
- 1 teaspoon olive oil
- 3 cups hot cooked whole wheat noodles
- Snipped parsley (optional)

Directions

1. Place chicken thighs 1 a 3 ½ or 4 quart slow cooker. In a large bowl stir together tomatoes, carrots, onion, broth, vinegar, rosemary, thyme and pepper. Pour over chicken in cooker.
2. Cover and cook on low heat setting for 8 to 10 hours.
3. Just before serving, in a large nonstick skillet cook and stir mushrooms in hot oil over medium-high heat for 8 to 10

minutes or until golden. Remove chicken from cooker. Remove chicken from bones; discard bones. Stir chicken and mushrooms into mixture in cooker. Serve chicken mixture over hot cooked noodles. If desired, sprinkle each serving with parsley.

Sage and Garlic Grilled Chicken Breasts

Ingredients:

- 1 teaspoon dried sage leaves
- ½ teaspoon seasoned salt
- ½ teaspoon dried marjoram leaves
- ¼ teaspoon coarse ground black pepper
- 2 garlic cloves, minced
- 2 tablespoons olive oil
- 4 boneless skinless chicken breast halves

Directions:

1. Heat closed contact grill for 5 minutes.
2. Meanwhile, in small bowl, combine all ingredients except chicken breast halves; mix well. Place chicken on sheet of waxed paper. Brush or rub mixture onto all sides of chicken.
3. When grill is heated, place chicken on bottom grill surface. Close grill; cook 5 to 7 minutes or until chicken is fork-tender and juices run clear.

Herb & Garlic Chicken with Vegetables

Ingredients:

- 1 cut-up whole chicken (3 to 3 1/2 lb)
- 2 tablespoons olive or vegetable oil

- 1 envelope savory herb with garlic soup mix (from 2.4-oz box)
- 1/3 cup chicken broth
- 4 medium stalks celery, cut in half lengthwise, then cut into 4-inch pieces
- 1 large onion, cut into 6 wedges
- 2 large carrots, cut in half lengthwise, then cut into 4-inch pieces
- 2 medium unpeeled russet potatoes, each cut into 8 pieces

Directions:

1. Heat oven to 425°F. Remove skin from chicken if desired. In small bowl, mix oil, soup mix and broth. Brush both sides of chicken pieces with about half of the oil mixture.
2. In large bowl, mix celery, onion, carrots, potatoes and remaining oil mixture. Arrange vegetables in ungreased 15x10x1-inch pan. Bake 15 minutes.
3. Place chicken pieces in pan, overlapping vegetables if necessary. Bake 35 to 40 minutes longer or until vegetables are tender and juice of chicken is clear when thickest piece is cut to bone (170°F for breasts; 180°F for thighs and legs).

Braised Chicken with Wild Mushrooms and Thyme

- 1 cup boiling water
- ½ oz dried porcini mushrooms
- 1 tablespoon butter
- 1 tablespoon olive oil
- 1 cut-up broiler-fryer chicken (3 to 3 1/2 lb)
- 2 large onions, chopped (2 cups)
- 5 cloves garlic, finely chopped
- 6 medium button mushrooms, sliced
- 2 medium carrots, chopped (1 cup)

- 2 medium stalks celery, chopped (1 cup)
- 2 dried bay leaves
- 2 fresh thyme sprigs or 1 teaspoon dried thyme leaves
- 5 tablespoons chopped fresh parsley
- 1 cup chicken broth
- ½ cup dry white wine or chicken broth
- 1 can (14.5 oz) diced tomatoes, undrained
- ¼ teaspoon salt
- ¼ teaspoon freshly ground pepper

Directions

1. Adjust oven rack to middle position. Heat oven to 300°F.
2. In small bowl, pour boiling water over dried mushrooms. Let stand 30 minutes to allow mushrooms to rehydrate (if mushrooms float to surface, place small saucer in bowl to keep them submerged). Use slotted spoon to remove rehydrated mushrooms from water; set aside. Reserve mushroom water.
3. In 4- or 5-quart ovenproof Dutch oven, heat butter and oil over medium-high heat until butter is melted. Add half of the chicken pieces and cook 6 minutes, turning occasionally, until chicken is deep golden brown (you are not cooking the chicken, just giving it color). Remove chicken from Dutch oven and place on plate. Repeat with remaining chicken.
4. Reduce heat to medium and add onions and garlic. Cook 5 minutes, stirring occasionally, until soft. Add rehydrated and sliced button mushrooms, carrots, celery, bay leaves, thyme and 3 tablespoons of the parsley. Cook 5 minutes, stirring occasionally, until vegetables are softened and mushrooms give up their juices.
5. Add reserved mushroom water and heat to a simmer. Simmer uncovered 10 minutes (you are trying to concentrate the flavor of the liquid). Add chicken (along with any juices

that may have accumulated on plate), broth, wine, tomatoes, salt and pepper.
6. Cover pan and place in oven. Bake 1 1/2 hours or until chicken is very tender and there is a good amount of broth. Remove and discard bay leaves and thyme sprig. Place 2 pieces chicken into each of 4 large, flat serving bowls and ladle broth over. Sprinkle with remaining 2 tablespoons parsley.

Asparagus Chicken Divan

Ingredients

- 1 pound skinless, boneless
- chicken breast halves
- 2 pounds fresh asparagus, trimmed
- 1 (10.75 ounce) can condensed cream of chicken soup, undiluted
- 1 teaspoon Worcestershire sauce
- ¼ teaspoon ground nutmeg
- 1 cup grated Parmesan cheese,
- ½ cup whipping cream, whipped
- ¾ cup mayonnaise*

Directions

1. Broil chicken 6 in. from the heat until juices run clear.
2. Meanwhile, in a large skillet, bring ½in. of water to a boil. Add asparagus. Reduce heat; cover and simmer for 3-5 minutes or until crisptender.
3. Drain and place in a greased shallow 2 ½-qt. baking dish. Cut chicken into thin slices. In a bowl, combine the soup, Worcestershire sauce and nutmeg. Spread half over asparagus.

Sprinkle with 1/3 cup Parmesan cheese. Top with chicken. Spread remaining soup mixture over chicken; sprinkle with 1/3 cup Parmesan cheese.
4. Bake, uncovered, at 400 degrees F for 20 minutes. Fold whipped cream into mayonnaise; spread over top. Sprinkle with remaining Parmesan cheese. Broil 4-6 in. from the heat for about 2 minutes or until golden brown.

Balsamic Chicken Breasts

Ingredients

- 2 sweet potatoes, peeled and cut into 2-inch pieces
- 1 tablespoon olive oil
- 2 skinless, boneless chicken breast halves
- ½ cup balsamic vinegar salt and ground black pepper for taste
- ½ cup balsamic vinegar

Directions

1. Preheat oven to 400 degrees F (200 degrees C).
2. Place the potatoes on a baking sheet; drizzle olive oil over potatoes and season with salt and pepper.
3. Place the chicken breasts in a baking dish. Pour 1/2 cup of balsamic vinegar over the breasts; season with salt and pepper. Cover with aluminum foil. Place the potatoes in the preheated oven and bake for 10 minutes; place the dish with the chicken in the oven and cook both the potatoes and chicken another 20 minutes; flip both the potatoes and chicken; reduce the oven heat to 350 degrees F (175 degrees C).
4. Bake another 20 minutes.

5. Pour 1/2 cup of balsamic vinegar into a small saucepan and place over medium heat. Cook until reduced to about 1/4 cup. Place the chicken breasts atop the potatoes; drizzle with the reduced balsamic vinegar to serve.

Caribbean-Spiced Roast Chicken

Ingredients

- 1 ½ tablespoons fresh lime juice
- 2 fluid ounces rum
- 1 tablespoon brown sugar
- ¼ teaspoon cayenne pepper
- ¼ teaspoon ground clove
- ½ teaspoon ground cinnamon
- ½ teaspoon ground ginger
- 1 teaspoon black pepper
- ½ teaspoon salt
- ½ teaspoon dried thyme leaves
- 1 (3 pound) whole chicken
- 1 tablespoon vegetable oil

Directions

1. Preheat oven to 325 degrees F (165 degrees C).
2. In a small bowl, combine the lime juice, rum, and brown sugar; set aside. Mix together the cayenne pepper, clove, cinnamon, ginger, pepper, salt, and thyme leaves. Brush the chicken with oil, then coat with the spice mixture.
3. Place in a roasting pan, and bake about 90 minutes, until the juices run clear or until a meat thermometer inserted in thickest part of the thigh reaches 180 degrees F. Baste the chicken with the sauce every 20 minutes while it's cooking. Allow chicken to rest for 10 minutes before carving.

Chapter 10: Turkey

Lime Turkey

Ingredients

- 2 turkey breast tenderloins 1 ½ pounds total
- ¼ finely snipped mint
- 2 teaspoons finely shredded lime peel
- ¼ cup lime juice
- 3 tablespoons orange juice
- 1 tablespoon olive oil
- 1 tablespoon honey
- ¼ teaspoon salt
- ¼ teaspoon black pepper
- 4 cut-up cups of cantaloupe
- Lime wedges
- Fresh mint sprigs (optional)

Directions

1. Cut each tenderloin in half horizontally to make four steaks. Place turkey steaks in a re-sealable plastic bag set in a shallow dish. For marinade, in a bowl whisk together mint, lime peel, lime juice, orange juice, olive oil, honey, salt and pepper. Reserve two tablespoons of marinade; cover and chill. Pour remaining marinade over turkey in bag; seal bag. Marinate in refrigerator for 4 to 6 hours, turning bag intermittently.
2. Drain turkey, discarding marinade. On a gas grill, set heat to medium and place turkey over heat. Grill, uncovered, for 12 to 15 minutes until no longer pink turning over once halfway through grilling.
3. Meanwhile, place cantaloupe in a bowl. Drizzle the 2 tablespoons reserved marinade over cantaloupe and toss to

coat. Serve turkey with cantaloupe and lime wedges. If you wish, you can garnish with the optional mint sprigs.

Grilled Turkey Kabobs

Ingredients

- 1/3 cup chili sauce
- 2 tablespoons lemon juice
- 1 tablespoon sugar
- 2 bay leaves
- 1 pound turkey breast tenderloins, cut into 1/2-inch cubes
- 2 medium zucchini, cut into 1/2 inch slices
- 2 small green peppers, cut into 1 1/2 inch squares
- 2 small onions, quartered
- 8 medium fresh mushrooms
- 8 cherry tomatoes
- 1 tablespoon canola oil

Directions

1. In a bowl, combine the chili sauce, lemon juice, sugar and bay leaves; mix well. Pour 1/4 cup marinade into a large resealable plastic bag; add the turkey. Seal bag and turn to coat; refrigerate for at least 2 hours or overnight. Cover and refrigerate remaining marinade.
2. Coat grill rack with nonstick cooking spray before starting the grill. Drain and discard marinade. Discard bay leaves from reserved marinade. On eight metal or soaked wooden skewers, alternately thread turkey and vegetables. Brush lightly with oil.
3. Grill, uncovered, over medium-hot heat for 3-4 minutes on each side or until juices run clear, basting frequently with reserved marinade and turning three times.

Grandma's Turkey Meatloaf

Ingredients

- 1 ½ pounds ground turkey
- 1 small onion, minced
- 2 stalks celery, minced
- 3 cloves garlic, minced
- 2 teaspoons chopped fresh basil
- ¼ cup Parmesan cheese
- ½ cup whole wheat bread crumbs
- 1 egg
- ¼ cup milk
- 1 (10.75 ounce) can condensed tomato soup

Directions

1. Preheat an oven to 350 degrees F (175 degrees C). Prepare a 9x13 inch baking dish with cooking spray.
2. Mix the ground turkey, onion, celery, garlic, basil, Parmesan cheese, bread crumbs, egg, and milk together in a large bowl. Shape the mixture into a loaf and place into prepared pan. Pour the tomato soup over the meatloaf. Cover tightly with aluminum foil.
3. Bake in the preheated oven until no longer pink in the center, about 45 minutes. An instant-read thermometer inserted into the center should read at least 165 degrees F (74 degrees C).

Caprese Turkey Burger

Ingredients

- 1 tablespoon balsamic vinegar
- 1 tablespoon extra virgin olive oil

- 4 thick slices tomato
- 1 1/3 pounds lean ground turkey
- 1 tablespoon tomato paste
- ¼ cup chopped fresh basil
- ¼ cup grated Parmesan cheese
- 1 clove garlic, minced
- ¼ teaspoon black pepper
- 4 ounces fresh mozzarella cheese, sliced
- 4 hamburger buns, split

Directions

1. Whisk the balsamic vinegar, oil, salt, and pepper in a small bowl. Pour over tomato slices to marinate.
2. Preheat an outdoor grill for medium-high heat, and lightly oil the grate.
3. Mix ground turkey, tomato paste, basil, Parmesan cheese, garlic, and 1I4 teaspoon pepper in a large bowl. Form beef mixture into 4 equal patties.
4. Cook on the preheated grill until the burgers are cooked to your desired degree of doneness, about 5 minutes per side for well done. An instant-read thermometer inserted into the center should read 160 degrees F (70 degrees C). Top each turkey burger with mozzarella cheese; allow to melt. Serve on hamburger buns with marinated tomato slices

Goat Cheese and Spinach Turkey Burgers

- 1 ½ pounds ground turkey breast
- 1cup frozen chopped spinach, thawed and drained
- 2 tablespoons goat cheese, crumbled
- 4 hamburger buns, split

Directions

1. Preheat the oven broiler.
2. In a medium bowl, mix ground turkey, spinach, and goat cheese. Form the mixture into 4 patties.
3. Arrange patties on a broiler pan, and place in the center of the preheated oven 15 minutes, or until done.

Spicy Turkey Burgers

Ingredients

- 2 pounds lean ground turkey
- 2 tablespoons minced garlic
- 1 teaspoon minced fresh ginger root
- 2 fresh green chile peppers, diced
- 1 medium red onion, diced
- ½ cup fresh cilantro, finely chopped
- 1 teaspoon salt
- ¼ cup low sodium soy sauce
- 1 tablespoon freshly ground black pepper
- 3 tablespoons paprika
- 1 tablespoon ground dry mustard
- 1 tablespoon ground cumin
- 1 dash Worcestershire sauce
- 4 hamburger buns, split

Directions

1. Preheat the grill for high heat.
2. In a bowl, mix the ground turkey, garlic, ginger, chile peppers, red onion, cilantro, salt, soy sauce, black pepper, paprika, mustard, cumin, and Worcestershire sauce. Form the mixture into 8 burger patties. Lightly oil the grill grate.

3. Place turkey burgers on the grill, and cook 5 to 10 minutes per side, until well done.

Grilled Turkey Tenderloins

Ingredients

- ¼ cup reduced-sodium soy sauce
- 4 teaspoons canola oil
- 1 teaspoon sugar
- 1 garlic clove, minced
- ½ teaspoon ground ginger
- ½ teaspoon ground mustard
- ¾ pound turkey breast tenderloins

Directions

1. In a bowl, combine the soy sauce, oil, sugar, garlic, ginger and mustard. Pour 1/4 cup marinade into a large re-sealable plastic bag; add the turkey. Seal bag and turn to coat; refrigerate for up to 4 hours. Cover and refrigerate remaining marinade for basting.
2. Coat grill rack with nonstick cooking spray before starting the grill. Drain and discard marinade from turkey. Grill turkey, covered, over medium heat for 8-10 minutes or until a meat thermometer reads 170 degrees F, turning twice and basting occasionally with reserved marinade. Cut into slices.

Turkey Steaks with Spinach, Pears and Blue Cheese

Ingredients

- 2 8 to 10 ounce turkey breast tenderloins

- 1 teaspoon of crushed dried sage
- ¼ teaspoon salt
- 1/8 teaspoon black pepper
- 2 tablespoons butter
- 1 6 ounce package of fresh baby spinach
- 1 large pear, cored and sliced thinly
- ¼ cup crumbled reduced-fat blue cheese

Directions

1. Split tenderloins horizontally to make four ½ inch thick steaks. Rub turkey with sage; springle with salt and pepper. In an extra large skillet, cook steaks in 1 tablespoon of the butter over medium -high heat for 14-16 minutes until no longer pink making sure to turn over once. Should turkey brown to quickly reduce the heat to medium. Remove turkey from skillet. Add spinach to skillet. Cook and stir until just wilted.
2. Meanwhile, in a small skillet cook pear slices in the remaining 1 tablespoon butter over medium to medium high heat, stirring occasionally, about 5 minutes or until tender and lightly browned.
3. Serve turkey steaks with spinach and pear slices. Sprinkle with the blue cheese.

Ginger-Orange Glazed Turkey Breasts

Ingredients

- 2 1 ½ pound skinless boneless turkey breasts
- 2 cloves garlic, cut into 12 slivers total
- 2 small fresh red chile peppers cut into 12 pieces
- ¼ cup orange juice
- ¼ cup olive oil
- 1 cup orange marmalade
- ½ cup finely chopped green onions (4)
- ½ cup orange juice

- 1 tablespoon grated fresh ginger
- 1 clove garlic, minced
- 1 tablespoon orange liqueur
- 1 teaspoon black pepper
- ½ teaspoon salt
- Sliced green onion, chopped chile peppers and finely shredded orange peel

Directions

1. Using a paring knife, cut 12 slits into the top or each turkey breast. Tuck a garlic sliver or chile pepper piece in to each slit, alternating garlic and chile pepper. Place turkey breast side by side in a a shallow glass baking dish.
2. In a small bowl combine the ¼ cup orange juice and the olive oil; pour over turkey. Cover; marinate in refrigerator for 12 to 24 hours, turning occasionally.
3. For the glaze, in a small saucepan combine the marmalade, green onions, the ½ cup orange juice, the ginger and minced garlic. Bring to boiling; reduce heat. Simmer, uncovered for 5 minutes. Remove from heat; stir in the orange liqueur.
4. Preheat oven to 350F. remove turkey breast from marinade; discard marinade. Arrange turkey breasts on a rack on a large roasting pan. Spoon some of the glaze over turkey breasts, being careful not to let the spoon touch the uncooked turkey. Sprinkle with black pepper and salt.
5. Roast for 45 to 50 minutes. Or until an instant read thermometer inserted into the thickest part of each breast reads 160F, spooning some of the remaining glaze over turkey breasts every 15 minutes of roasting, each time being careful not to let the spoon touch the uncooked turkey. Let turkey stand for 5 minutes before slicing. If desired, , garnish with additional sliced onion, chopped chile peppers and finely shredded orange peel.

Chapter 11: Fish

Grilled Tuna Steaks

Ingredients

- 8 (3 ounce) fillets fresh tuna steaks, 1 inch thick
- ½ cup soy sauce
- 1/3 cup sherry
- ¼ cup Olive oil
- 1 tablespoon fresh lime juice
- 1 clove garlic, minced

Directions

1. Place tuna steaks in a shallow baking dish. In a medium bowl, mix soy sauce, sherry, olive oil, fresh lime juice, and garlic. Pour the soy sauce mixture over the tuna steaks, and turn to coat. Cover, and refrigerate for at least one hour.
2. Preheat grill for high heat. Lightly oil grill grate.
3. Place tuna steaks on grill, and discard remaining marinade. Grill for 3 to 6 minutes per side, or to your preference.

Lemony Halibut

Instructions

- 6 (6 ounce) fillets halibut
- 3 teaspoons dried dill weed
- 3 teaspoons onion powder
- ¼ teaspoon paprika seasoning
- salt to taste
- 1 pinch lemon pepper

- 2 teaspoons dried parsley
- 1 pinch garlic powder
- 2 tablespoons lemon juice

Directions

1. Preheat oven to 375 degrees F (190 degrees C). Cut 6 foil squares, large enough for the size of each fillet. Center fillets on the foil squares and sprinkle each with dill weed, onion powder, paprika, seasoned salt, lemon pepper, parsley and garlic powder.
2. Sprinkle lemon juice over each fillet. Fold foil over fillets to make a pocket. Pleat seams to securely enclose.
3. Place packets on a baking sheet and bake in the preheat oven for 30 minutes.

Pepper Crust Salmon with Yogurt-Lime Sauce

Ingredients

- 4 4 to 5 ounce skinless salmon fillets
- ½ teaspoon multi-colored peppercorns, crushed
- ¼ teaspoon salt
- 2 teaspoons olive oil
- ¾ cup plain non-fat yogurt
- 1 tablespoon honey
- 1 tablespoon snipped fresh parsley
- ¼ teaspoon shredded lime peel
- 2 teaspoons lime juice
- ½ teaspoon minced fresh ginger
- Lime peels and parsley leaves are optional

Directions

1. Sprinkle salmon with peppercorns and salt; gently press peppercorns into the salmon. In a large nonstick skillet heat oil over medium-high heat. Add salmon; cook for 3 minutes more or until fish flakes easily when tested with a fork.
2. Meanwhile, in a medium bowl, combine yogurt, honey, snipped pasley, finely shredded lime peel, lime juice and ginger.
3. Serve salmon with yogurt-lime sauce.

Tilapia Fish Tacos

Ingredients

- 1 cup of corn
- ½ cup diced red onion
- 1 cup peeled, chopped jicama
- ½ cup diced red bell pepper
- 1 cup fresh cilantro leaves
- finely chopped 1 lime, zested and juiced
- 2 tablespoons sour cream
- 2 tablespoons cayenne pepper
- 1 tablespoon ground black pepper
- 2 tablespoons salt
- 6 (4 ounce) fillets tilapia
- 2 tablespoons olive oil
- 12 corn tortillas, warmed

Directions

1. Preheat grill for high heat. In a medium bowl, mix together corn, red onion, jicama, red bell pepper, and cilantro. Stir in lime juice and zest.
2. In a small bowl, combine cayenne pepper, ground black pepper, and salt.

3. Brush each fillet with olive oil, and sprinkle with spices.
4. Arrange fillets on grill grate, and cook for 3 minutes per side. For each fiery fish taco, top two corn tortillas with fish, sour cream, and corn salsa.

Rainbow Trout Cooked in Foil

Ingredients

- 2 rainbow trout fillets
- 1 tablespoon olive oil
- 2 teaspoons garlic salt
- 1 teaspoon ground black pepper
- 1 fresh jalapeno pepper
- 1 lemon, sliced

Directions

1. Preheat oven to 400 degrees F (200 degrees C). Rinse fish, and pat dry. Rub fillets with olive oil, and season with garlic salt and black pepper.
2. Place each fillet on a large sheet of aluminum foil. Top with jalapeno slices, and squeeze the juice from the ends of the lemons over the fish. Arrange lemon slices on top of fillets. Carefully seal all edges of the foil to form enclosed packets. Place packets on baking sheet.
3. Bake in preheated oven for 15 to 20 minutes, depending on the size of fish. Fish is done when it flakes easily with a fork.

Grilled Lemon Garlic Halibut Steaks

Ingredients

- ¼ cup lemon juice

- 1 tablespoon vegetable oil
- ¼ teaspoon salt
- ¼ teaspoon pepper
- 2 cloves garlic, finely chopped
- 4 halibut or tuna steaks, about 1 inch thick (about 2 pounds)
- ¼ cup chopped fresh parsley
- 1 tablespoon grated lemon peel

Directions

1. Brush grill rack with vegetable oil. Heat coals or gas grill for direct heat. In shallow glass or plastic dish or resealable food-storage plastic bag, mix lemon juice, 1 tablespoon oil, the salt, pepper and garlic. Add fish; turn several times to coat with marinade. Cover dish or seal bag and refrigerate 10 minutes.
2. Remove fish from marinade; reserve marinade. Cover and grill fish 4 to 6 inches from medium heat 10 to 15 minutes, turning once and brushing with marinade, until fish flakes easily with fork. Discard any remaining marinade.
3. Sprinkle fish with parsley and lemon peel.

Sicilian Tuna with Capers

Ingredients

- 4 fresh or frozen tuna steaks, cut 1 inch thick (about 1 pound total)
- 2 tablespoons red wine vinegar
- 1 tablespoon snipped fresh dill weed or 1 teaspoon dried dill weed
- 2 teaspoons olive oil
- ¼ teaspoon salt
- 1/8 teaspoon cayenne pepper

- ½ cup chopped tomato
- 1 tablespoon capers, drained
- 1 tablespoon chopped pitted ripe olives
- 1 clove garlic, minced
- Hot cooked rice (optional)
- Steamed baby bok choy (optional)

Directions

1. Preheat broiler. Thaw fish, if frozen. Rinse fish and pat dry with paper towels. For marinade, in a shallow dish combine vinegar, dill weed, oil salt and half of the cayenne pepper. Add fish to marinade in dish, turning to coat. Cover and marinate in the refrigerator for 15 minutes.
2. Meanwhile, in a small bowl stir together tomatoes, capers, olives, garlic and the remaining cayenne pepper.
3. Drain fish, reserving marinade. Place fish on the greased unheated rack of a broiler pan. Broil 4 inches from the heat for 4 minutes. Turn fish and brush with all the reserved marinade. Broil for 4 to 8 minutes more or until fish begins to flake when tested with a fork. Serve tuna topped with tomato mixture. If desired, serve over hot cooked rice with steamed baby bok choy.

Tuna with Sweet & Heat Salsa

Ingredients

- 2 5 ounce fresh or frozen tuna steaks, cut ¾ to 1 inch thick
- ½ teaspoon cumin seeds
- ½ teaspoon finely shredded lime peel
- 2 tablespoons lime juice
- 1 tablespoon canola oil
- ½ teaspoon crushed red pepper
- ½ teaspoon salt

- 1 recipe Sweet & Heat Salsa
- Lime wedges (optional)

Directions

1. Thaw fish, if frozen. Rinse fish; pat dry. Place fish in large resealable plastic bag. Set aside. In a small dry skillet heat cumin seeds over medium heat 1 to 2 minutes or until you smell the aroma, shaking skillet occasionally. Crush cumin seeds in a mortar and pestle.
2. Combine crushed cumin seeds, the lime peel, lime juice, oil, crushed red pepper and salt. Pour over fish in bag; turn to coat fish. Seal bag. Marinate in the refrigerator for 30 to 60 minutes, turning the bag every so often.
3. Prepare Sweet & heat Salsa; set aside. Drain fish, discarding marinade. For charcoal grill, place fish on the greased grill rack directly over medium coals. Grill, uncovered for 6 to 10 minutes or until fish flakes easily, gently turning once halfway through grilling. (For a gas grill, preheat grill. Reduce heat to medium. Place fish on greased grill rack over heat. Cover and grill as directed.) Serve fish topped with salsa. If you wish, you may use the lime wedges.

Roasted Salmon and Vegetables

Ingredients:

- 4 salmon steaks, ½ inch thick (about 1 ½ lb)
- 2 cups refrigerated new potato wedges with skins (from 20-oz bag)
- 2 small zucchini, quartered lengthwise, then cut into 2-inch pieces
- 1 medium red bell pepper, cut into 2-inch pieces
- 1 tablespoon lemon juice

- 1 tablespoon butter or margarine, melted
- ½ teaspoon salt
- ¼ to ½ teaspoon dried tarragon leaves
- ¼ teaspoon pepper

Directions:

1. Heat oven to 425°F. Place salmon steaks in ungreased 15x10x1-inch pan. Arrange potato wedges, zucchini and bell pepper around salmon.
2. Brush salmon with lemon juice. Brush salmon and vegetables with butter; sprinkle with salt, tarragon and pepper.
3. Bake 25 to 35 minutes or until salmon flakes easily with fork and vegetables are tender.

Chapter 12: Meatless

Mac & Cheese

Ingredients

- 1 tablespoon vegetable oil
- 1 tablespoon butter
- 1 teaspoon garlic and parsley powder
- 1 teaspoon onion powder
- 1 tablespoon sriracha sauce
- 1 cup low or no sodium chicken bouillon
- ½ cup low fat milk
- 1 8 oz. box elbow macaroni
- 1 cup Monterey Jack cheese
- ½ cups plain bread crumbs

Directions

1. Place in the bottom of the crockpot: olive oil, butter, garlic powder and parsley, onion powder, sriracha sauce chicken bouillon, and milk
2. Pour in the macaroni and cheese and stir well.
3. Cook 1 ½ hours on low. Thirty minutes before it's done top with the bread crumbs.

Pasta and Pepper Primavera

Ingredients

- 4 ounces dried multigrain spaghetti
- 2 teaspoons bottled minced garlic or 4 cloves garlic, minced
- 1 tablespoon olive oil

- 1 16 ounce package of frozen peppers and onion mix or stir fry vegetable mix
- 1 15 ounce can cannellini beans, rinsed and drained
- ¼ cup dry white wine or reduced sodium chicken broth
- ½ teaspoon finely shredded lemon peel (set aside)
- 1 tablespoon lemon juice
- ½ teaspoon dried thyme, crushed
- ¼ teaspoon salt
- ¼ freshly ground black pepper
- ¼ teaspoon crushed red pepper
- 1 tablespoon butter
- 1 ounce Parmesan cheese, shaved

Directions

1. Cook pasta as directed on the package.
2. Meanwhile, in a large skillet cook and stir garlic in hot oil over medium heat for 30 seconds. Add frozen vegetables. Cook and stir for 2 minutes. Add beans, wine, lemon juice, thyme, salt, black pepper and crushed red pepper. Bring to boiling; reduce heat. Cook, uncovered, about 4 minutes or until vegetables are crisp tender, stirring occasionally. Remove from heat. Stir in butter.
3. Drain pasta. Add pasta to vegetable mixture in skillet. Toss gently to combine.
4. Divide pasta mixture among four shallow bowls. Sprinkle with Parmesan and lemon peel. Serve.

Chile

Ingredients:

- 2 medium unpeeled white or red potatoes (about 10 oz), cut into 1/2-inch cubes
- 1 medium onion, chopped (1/2 cup)

- 1 small bell pepper (any color), chopped (1/2 cup)
- 1 can (15 oz) chickpeas (garbanzo beans), drained, rinsed
- 1 can (15 oz) kidney beans, drained, rinsed
- 2 cans (14.5 oz each) organic diced tomatoes, undrained
- 1 can (8 oz) organic tomato sauce
- 1 tablespoon chili powder
- 1 teaspoon ground cumin
- 1 medium zucchini, cut into 1/2-inch slices

Directions:

1. In 4-quart Dutch oven, place all ingredients except zucchini; stir well. Heat to boiling over high heat, stirring occasionally; reduce heat. Cover; simmer 10 minutes.
2. Stir in zucchini. Cover; cook 5 to 7 minutes longer, stirring occasionally, until potatoes and zucchini are tender when pierced with fork.

Oven-Roasted Potatoes and Vegetables

Ingredients:

- 2 ½ cups refrigerated new potato wedges (from 1 lb 4-oz bag)
- 1 medium red bell pepper, cut into 1-inch pieces
- 1 small zucchini, cut into 1/2-inch pieces
- 4 oz fresh whole mushrooms, quartered (about 1 cup)
- 2 teaspoons olive oil
- ½ teaspoon dried Italian seasoning
- ¼ teaspoon garlic salt

Directions:

1. Heat oven to 450°F. Spray 15x10x1-inch pan with cooking spray. In large bowl, toss all ingredients to coat. Spread evenly in pan.
2. Bake 15 to 20 minutes, stirring once halfway through baking time, until vegetables are tender and lightly browned.

Zucchini Spaghetti

Ingredients:

- 6 oz uncooked spaghetti
- 3 cups chopped zucchini (2 medium)
- 1/3 cup water
- 1 tablespoon tomato paste
- ¼ teaspoon kosher (coarse) salt
- 1/8 teaspoon coarse ground black pepper
- 1 can (15.5 oz) great northern beans, drained, rinsed
- 1 can (14.5 oz) diced tomatoes with basil, garlic and oregano, undrained
- ½ cup crumbled feta cheese (2 oz)

Directions:

1. Cook spaghetti as directed on package, omitting salt and oil; drain.
2. Meanwhile, spray 12-inch skillet with olive oil cooking spray; heat over medium-high heat. Add zucchini; cook 5 minutes, stirring occasionally, until lightly browned. Stir in water, tomato paste, salt, pepper, beans and tomatoes. Cover; simmer 4 minutes or until thoroughly heated.
3. On each of 4 plates, place about 2/3 cup spaghetti. Top each with 1 cup zucchini mixture and 2 tablespoons cheese.

Roasted Rosemary-Onion Potatoes

Ingredients:

- 4 medium potatoes (1 1/3 pounds)
- 1 small onion, finely chopped (1/4 cup)
- 2 tablespoons olive or vegetable oil
- 2 tablespoons chopped fresh rosemary leaves or 2 teaspoons dried rosemary leaves
- 1 teaspoon chopped fresh thyme leaves or 1/4 teaspoon dried thyme leaves
- ¼ teaspoon salt
- 1/8 teaspoon pepper

Directions:

1. Heat oven to 450ºF. Grease jelly roll pan, 15 1/2x10 1/2x1 inch. Cut potatoes into 1-inch chunks.
2. Mix remaining ingredients in large bowl. Add potatoes; toss to coat. Spread potatoes in single layer in pan.
3. Bake uncovered 20 to 25 minutes, turning occasionally, until potatoes are light brown and tender when pierced with fork.

Lasagna Primavera

Ingredients

- 12 uncooked lasagna noodles
- 3 cups frozen broccoli cuts, thawed and well drained
- 3 large carrots, coarsely shredded (2 cups)
- 2 cups organic diced tomatoes (from 28-oz can), well drained
- 2 medium bell peppers, cut into ½-inch pieces
- 1 container (15 oz) ricotta cheese
- ½ cup grated Parmesan cheese
- 1 egg

- 2 containers (10 oz each) refrigerated Alfredo pasta sauce
- 1 package (16 oz) shredded mozzarella cheese (4 cups)

Directions

1. Heat oven to 350°F. Cook and drain noodles as directed on package.
2. Meanwhile, if necessary, cut broccoli florets into bite-size pieces. In large bowl, mix broccoli, carrots, tomatoes and bell peppers. In small bowl, mix ricotta cheese, Parmesan cheese and egg.
3. In ungreased 13x9-inch (3-quart) glass baking dish, spread 2/3 cup Alfredo sauce. Top with 4 noodles. Spread half of the cheese mixture and 2 ½ cups of the vegetables over noodles. Spoon 2/3 cup sauce in dollops over vegetables. Sprinkle with 1 cup of the mozzarella cheese.
4. Top with 4 noodles; spread with remaining cheese mixture and 2 ½ cups of vegetables. Spoon 2/3 cup sauce in dollops over vegetables. Sprinkle with 1 cup mozzarella cheese. Top with remaining 4 noodles and the vegetables. Spoon remaining
sauce in dollops over vegetables. Sprinkle with remaining 2 cups mozzarella cheese.
5. Bake uncovered 45 to 60 minutes or until bubbly and hot in center. Let stand 15 minutes before cutting.

Chiles Rellenos

Ingredients

- 2 large fresh poblano chile peppers, Anaheim chile peppers or green sweet peppers (8 ounces)
- 1 cup shredded reduced-fat Mexican-style cheese blend (4 ounces)

- 1 or 2 fresh jalapeno chile peppers, seeded and finely chopped
- 1 ½ cups of refrigerated frozen egg product, thawed or eggs beaten
- ½ cup fat free milk
- ½ cup flour
- ½ teaspoon baking powder
- ¼ teaspoon cayenne pepper
- Picante sauce and light sour cream (optional)

Directions

1. Preheat oven to 450F. halve the poblano, Anaheim or sweet peppers and remove stems, ribs and seeds. Immerse peppers in boiling water for 3 minutes; drain. Invert peppers onto papers towels to drain well. Place one pepper half in each of the four greased 12 to 16 ounce au gratin dishes. Top each with cheese and jalapeno peppers.
2. In a medium bowl combine egg and milk. Add flour, baking powder and cayenne pepper. Beat until smooth. Pour egg mixture evenly over peppers and cheese in dishes.
3. Bake, uncovered for about 15 minutes or until a knife inserted into the egg mixture comes out clean. Let stand for about 5 minutes. If desired serve with the picante sauce and/ or sour cream.

Butternut Squash & Quinoa Pilaf

Ingredients

- 4 cups peeled and cubed butternut squash
- 6 cloves garlic, minced
- 1/8 teaspoon crushed red pepper
- 5 teaspoons olive oil
- ¼ cup sliced almonds
- 2 cups cooked quinoa
- 1 tablespoon snipped fresh sage

- ½ teaspoon salt

Directions

1. Preheat oven to 425F. In a large bowl, combine butternut squash, garlic and crushed red pepper. Drizzle with 2 teaspoons of the oil. Stir until squash is evenly coated. Spoon into a 15x10x1-inch baking pan. Roast 30 minutes, stirring once and adding the sliced almonds for the last 5 minutes of roasting.
2. In a large bowl, combine the quinoa, the remaining 3 teaspoons of oil, the snipped sage and salt. Stir in roasted squash and almonds. If desired, garnish with sage leaves.

Chapter 13: Desserts

Vanilla Bean Pudding

Ingredients

- 2 ½ cups
- 2% reduced-fat milk
- 1 vanilla bean, split lengthwise
- ¾ cup sugar
- 3 tablespoons cornstarch
- 1/8 teaspoon salt
- ¼ cup half-and-half
- 2 large egg yolks
- 4 teaspoons butter

Directions

1. Place milk in a medium, heavy saucepan. Scrape seeds from vanilla bean; add seeds and bean to milk. Bring to a boil.
2. Combine sugar, cornstarch, and salt in a large bowl, stirring well. Combine half-and-half and egg yolks, stirring well. Stir egg yolk mixture into sugar mixture. Gradually add half of hot milk to sugar mixture, stirring constantly with a whisk. Return hot milk mixture to pan; bring to a boil. Cook 1 minute, stirring constantly with a whisk. Remove from heat. Add butter, stirring until melted. Remove vanilla bean; discard.
3. Spoon pudding into a bowl. Place bowl in a large ice-filled bowl for 15 minutes or until pudding cools, stirring occasionally. Cover surface of pudding with plastic wrap; chill.

Strawberry and Peach Cream Trifle

Ingredients

- 2 packages (4-serving size each) vanilla pudding and pie filling mix, (not instant)
- 3 cups milk
- 1 ½ quarts (6 cups) strawberries, sliced
- 1 large fresh peach, peeled and cubed
- ¼ cup sugar
- 1 package (16 ounces) frozen pound cake loaf
- ¼ cup peach or strawberry preserves
- ¼ cup amaretto or orange juice
- 1 cup whipping (heavy) cream
- ¼ cup slivered almonds, toasted
- 2 large fresh peaches, peeled and sliced

Directions

1. Make pudding mix as directed on package for pudding, using 3 cups milk. Place plastic wrap directly on top of pudding. Refrigerate at least 2 hours until chilled.
2. Mix strawberries, cubed peach and sugar. Let stand at room temperature 15 minutes.
3. Cut pound cake horizontally in half. Spread preserves over bottom half. Top with top half. Cut into 18 slices. Drizzle with amaretto. Place 9 slices in 3- to 4-quart straight-sided glass bowl. Spoon half of strawberry mixture over cake.
4. Beat whipping cream in chilled small bowl with electric mixer on high speed until stiff. Fold whipped cream into pudding. Spoon half of pudding mixture over strawberries. Repeat layers with remaining cake, strawberry mixture and pudding mixture. Refrigerate at least 2 hours.
5. Just before serving, sprinkle with almonds. Top with sliced peaches.

Baked Apples w/ Walnuts & Honey

Ingredients

- 4 medium sized apples
- 1 cup finely chopped walnuts
- 1 tablespoon honey
- 1 egg white
- 1 teaspoon vanilla extract
- zest of a half of lemon
- pinch of salt

Directions

1. Preheat the oven at 350 degrees F.
2. Whip the egg white with the salt. the salt to stiff peaks, add the honey and beat until mixed. Fold in lemon zest, vanilla and walnuts.
3. Cut apples in pieces and core them. Lay the apples skin side down on a baking dish and fill the middle with the mixture. Bake for 40-45 minutes until apples are soft and filling crisps on top. Serve immediately.

Carrot-Pineapple Muffins

Ingredients

- 2 cups almond flour
- 2 whisked eggs
- 1 tablespoon coconut flour
- ½ cup peeled grated carrots
- ¾ cup chopped fresh pineapple
- ¼ cup melted raw honey
- ¼ cup melted coconut oil
- 1 teaspoon cinnamon
- ½ teaspoon baking soda
- ½ teaspoon sea salt

- ¼ teaspoon allspice
- 1/8 teaspoon cloves

Directions

1. Preheat the oven at 350 degrees.
2. In a mixing bowl combine dry ingredients. In another mixing bowl combine wet ingredients. Add wet ingredients to dry And stir until combined.
3. Bake for 40-45 minutes until apples are soft and filling crisps on top. Serve immediately.

Banana Bread

Ingredients

- 2 cups almond flour
- 2 tablespoons coconut flour
- 2 whisked eggs (include yolk)
- 3 mashed ripe bananas
- ¼ cup melted raw honey
- ¼ cup melted coconut oil
- 1 teaspoon vanilla extract
- 1 teaspoon cinnamon
- ¾ teaspoon baking soda
- ½ teaspoon sea salt

Directions

1. Preheat the oven at 350 degrees.
2. In mixing bowl combine dry ingredients (Almond flour, coconut flour, spices, baking soda and sea salt). In another bowl combine wet ingredients (eggs, honey, coconut oil,

vanilla extract). Add wet ingredients to dry ingredients and stir until combined. Add mashed bananas and mix together.
3. Place in a greased (non-stick cooking spray 9x5 loaf pan) and bake 40- 45 min depending on oven.

Raspberry Tarts

Ingredients

- 1 cup/ 250 ml milk
- ½ vanilla bean, halved lengthwise and seeds scraped
- 3 egg yolks
- ¼ cup/ 55 g sugar
- 2 tablespoons flour
- 1 tablespoon framboise (raspberry liqueur)
- ¼ cup/ 60 ml heavy cream
- 1 pound/ 450 g fresh raspberries
- 1 (9-inch/ 23 cm) prepared baked cookie crust

Directions

1. Put the milk in a saucepan. Split the vanilla bean, scraping the seeds into the milk, then drop in the pot. Heat to a simmer, remove from heat, cover, and set to infuse 10 minutes.
2. In bowl using an electric mixer, beat the yolks with the sugar until pale. Beat in the flour. Pull the vanilla bean from the milk and whisk the milk gradually into the egg mixture. Pour back into the saucepan, bring to a boil, and cook 1 minute. Remove from the heat and stir in the framboise. Strain into a bowl, cover with plastic wrap, and set aside to cool. When chilled, whip the cream and gently fold it in.
3. Spread the pastry cream evenly in the base of the prepared cookie crust. Arrange the berries neatly over top.

Apple-Nut Wedges

Ingredients

- Nonstick cooking spray
- 1 egg
- 2 egg whites
- 2/3 cup brown sugar
- 1 teaspoon vanilla
- 1/3 cup flour
- ¾ teaspoon baking soda
- 1/8 teaspoon salt
- 2 large apples, cored and chopped (2 cups)
- ½ cup chopped walnuts or pecans, toasted
- ½ cup light sour cream
- ¼ cup vanilla low-fat yogurt sweetened with artificial sweetener
- ½ teaspoon vanilla

Directions

1. Preheat oven to 325F. Coat a 9 inch pie plate with cooking spray; set aside.
2. In a large bowl, combine egg, egg whites, brown sugar and one teaspoon of vanilla. Beat with electric mixer on medium spread about 1 minute or until smooth. In a small bowl, stir together flour, baking soda and salt. Add flour mixture to the egg mixture; stir just until combined. Fold in apples and nuts. Spread batter evenly in the prepared pie plate.
3. Bake for 25 to 30 minutes or until center is set. Cool slightly on wire rack. Meanwhile, for topping, in a small bowl whisk to together sour cream, yogurt and the ½ teaspoon vanilla.
4. To serve, cut dessert into eight wedges. Serve warm. Spoon about 1 rounded tablespoon of the topping over each serving.

Fruit Popsicles with Coconut and Pineapple

Ingredients

- ¼ teaspoon salt
- ½ (14 ounce) can sweetened condensed milk
- ½ cup shredded coconut 1/2 cup minced pineapple
- ¼ teaspoon vanilla extract
- 1 (14 ounce) can coconut milk
- ¾ cup half-and-half

Directions

1. Combine all the ingredients except shredded coconut and pineapple pieces in a bowl. Stir in shredded coconut and pineapple; pour into ice-pop molds and make sure the fruit is arranged nicely. Put it in the freezer for at least 6 hours.
2. To remove from the molds, place for a few seconds under warm water. Serve.

Coffee Custard

Ingredients

- 1 envelope unflavored gelatin
- 2 cups fat-free milk
- 3 egg yolks
- ½ cup of sugar
- 1 ½ teaspoon vanilla
- 1 ½ teaspoons instant espresso coffee powder
- Frozen light whipped dessert topping (optional)
- Ground cinnamon (optional)

Directions

1. In a small bowl sprinkle gelatin over ¼ cup of the milk. Let stand for 5 minutes. Meanwhile, in a a medium saucepan

whisk together egg yolks and sugar. Gradually mix in the remain 1 ¾ cups milk. Cook and stir over medium heat. Gradually whisk about ½ cup of the hot milk mixture into the gelatin mixture. Whisk gelatin mixture into remaining milk mixture in saucepan. Place saucepan in large bowl of ice water. Stir in vanilla. Stir for a few minutes to cool the mixture. Remove ½ cup of the mixture to a small bowl. Stir in espresso powder until incorporated and dissolved. Cover and set espresso mixture aside.
2. Pour remaining mixture into four 6 ounce individual dishes, custard cups or glasses. Cover dishes; chill for 15 to 20 minutes. Drizzle the espresso mixture over the custard mixture in dishes. Using a thin metal spatula, lightly swirl the espresso mixture into the top of the custard. Cover dishes loosely and chill for 4 hours until set. If you wish, top with a little dessert topping and sprinkle some cinnamon over.

Creamy Fruit Tarts

Ingredients:

- 1 cup Bisquick mix
- 2 tablespoons sugar
- 1 tablespoon butter or margarine, softened
- 2 packages (3 ounces each) cream cheese, softened
- ¼ cup sugar
- ¼ cup sour cream
- 1 ½ cups assorted sliced fresh fruit or berries
- 1/3 cup apple jelly, melted

Directions:

1. Heat oven to 375°F. Mix Bisquick, 2 tablespoons sugar, the butter and 1 package cream cheese in small bowl until dough forms a ball.

2. Divide dough into 6 parts. Press each part dough on bottom and ¾ inch up side in each of 6 tart pans, 4 ¼ x 1 inch, or 10-ounce custard cups. Place on cookie sheet.
3. Bake 10 to 12 minutes or until light brown. Cool in pans on wire rack, about 30 minutes. Remove tart shells from pans.
4. Beat remaining package cream cheese, ¼ cup sugar and the sour cream until smooth. Spoon into tart shells, spreading over bottoms. Top each with about ¼ cup fruit. Brush with jelly.

Conclusion:

I had a lot of goals when I set out to write this book, but the most important of these was to shed light on gout and how to prevent it through a proper diet. As I am sure you've found, there are no shortage of great recipes out there to satisfy your taste buds.

You have one life to live. If you have gout, it is not a death sentence, but rather, a wake-up call for you to take better care of yourself. Think of it as a blessing in disguise. You are going to have to make some changes. That's it.

Whether you need to take medicine for it or not you should ensure that you follow these simple rules of thumb:

- Limit alcoholic beverages and drinks sweetened with fruit sugar (fructose).
- Drink plenty of nonalcoholic beverages, especially water.
- Limit intake of foods high in purines, such as red meat, organ meats and seafood.
- Exercise regularly and lose weight. Keeping your body at a healthy weight reduces your risk of gout.

I hope you enjoyed this book and found it useful. Now that you have a basic understanding of gout and its causes and remedies, I want you to act on what you have learned and BEAT gout into your past, where it belongs.

WITHDRAWN
from St. Joseph County Public Library
Excess __X__ Damaged _____
Date _10/19/21_ Initials _____

88496672R00050

Made in the USA
Columbia, SC
01 February 2018